Hyatt's Interpretation of Pulmonary Function Tests
A PRACTICAL GUIDE

FIFTH EDITION

Paul D. Scanlon, MD
Consultant
Division of Pulmonary and Critical Care Medicine
Mayo Clinic
Professor of Medicine
Mayo Clinic College of Medicine
Rochester, Minnesota

Robert E. Hyatt, MD
Emeritus Consultant (Deceased)
Division of Pulmonary and Critical Care Medicine
Mayo Clinic
Emeritus Professor of Medicine and Physiology
Mayo Clinic College of Medicine
Rochester, Minnesota

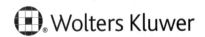. Wolters Kluwer

Philadelphia • Baltimore • New York • London
Buenos Aires • Hong Kong • Sydney • Tokyo

Acquisitions Editor: Robin Najar
Development Editor: Eric McDermott
Editorial Coordinator: Blair Jackson
Marketing Manager: Stacy Maylil
Production Project Manager: David Saltzberg
Design Coordinator: Holly Reid McLaughlin
Manufacturing Coordinator: Beth Welsh
Prepress Vendor: S4Carlisle Publishing Services
Cover illustration used with permission of Mayo Foundation for Medical Education and Research; all rights reserved.

Library of Congress Cataloging-in-Publication Data

Names: Hyatt, Robert E., author. | Scanlon, Paul D. (Paul David) author. |
   Hyatt, Robert E., author.
Title: Hyatt's interpretation of pulmonary function tests : a practical guide
   / Paul D. Scanlon, MD, Consultant, Division of Pulmonary and Critical Care
   Medicine, Mayo Clinic, Rochester, Minnesota; Professor of Medicine, Mayo
   Clinic College of Medicine, Rochester, Minnesota, Robert E. Hyatt, MD
   Emeritus Consultant (deceased), Division of Pulmonary and Critical Care
   Medicine Mayo Clinic, Rochester, Minnesota; Emeritus Professor of Medicine
   and of Physiology Mayo Clinic College of Medicine, Rochester, Minnesota.
Other titles: Interpretation of pulmonary function tests
Description: Fifth edition. | Philadelphia : Wolters Kluwer, 2020. | Revision
   of: Interpretation of pulmonary function tests. 2014. Fourth edition. |
   Includes bibliographical references and index.
Identifiers: LCCN 2019014824 | ISBN 9781975114343
Subjects: LCSH: Pulmonary function tests.
Classification: LCC RC734.P84 H93 2020 | DDC 616.2/40754—dc23 LC record available at https://
lccn.loc.gov/2019014824

shop.lww.com

Acknowledgments

Thanks to Lisa R. Gilbertson for her secretarial contributions. Without the help of Kenna Atherton, Jane M. Craig, and Leann Stee in the Section of Scientific Publications, this book would not have reached fruition. Thanks to Dr. Hyatt's children, Drs. Amanda Hyatt and Mark C. Hyatt for their continued support. Special thanks go to our pulmonary function technicians for their excellent work. Lastly, thanks to my wife, Maggie, for her support and for her nearly infinite patience.

About the Cover: The cartoon images depict the two main pathologic processes that contribute to airflow limitation in COPD. The development of emphysema, on the left, contributes to loss of elastic recoil, which is the main driving pressure for expiratory airflow. On the right, airway smooth muscle contraction, airway wall thickening due to inflammation, and mucous hypersecretion all contribute to airway narrowing, which increases airflow resistance. The flow–volume curve depicts central airflow limitation affecting both inspiratory and expiratory flow, but more severely limiting inspiratory flow and therefore likely extrathoracic, or upper airway, in location.

List of Abbreviations

$(A-a)\,D_{O_2}$	difference between the oxygen tensions of alveolar gas and arterial blood
BMI	body mass index
Ca_{O_2}	arterial oxygen-carrying capacity
C_{CW}	chest wall compliance
C_L	compliance of the lung
$C_{L_{dyn}}$	dynamic compliance of the lung
$C_{L_{stat}}$	static compliance of the lung
COHb	carboxyhemoglobin
COPD	chronic obstructive pulmonary disease
Crs	static compliance of entire respiratory system
D_L	diffusing capacity of the lungs
$D_{L_{CO}}$	diffusing capacity of carbon monoxide
$D_{L_{O_2}}$	diffusing capacity of oxygen
ERV	expiratory reserve volume
F	female
FEF	forced expiratory flow
FEF_{25}	forced expiratory flow after 25% of the FVC has been exhaled
FEF_{25-75}	forced expiratory flow over the middle 50% of the FVC
FEF_{50}	forced expiratory flow after 50% of the FVC has been exhaled
FEF_{75}	forced expiratory flow after 75% of the FVC has been exhaled
FEFmax	maximal forced expiratory flow
FEV_1	forced expiratory volume in 1 second
FEV_6	forced expiratory volume in 6 seconds
FEV_1/FVC	ratio of FEV_1 to the FVC
FIF_{50}	forced inspiratory flow after 50% of the FVC has been inhaled
$F_{I_{O_2}}$	fraction of inspired oxygen
FRC	functional residual capacity
FV	flow–volume

FVC	forced expiratory vital capacity
Hb	hemoglobin
IVC	inspiratory vital capacity
Kco	carbon monoxide transfer coefficient
LLN	lower limit normal
M	male
MetHb	methemoglobin
MFSR	maximal flow static recoil (curve)
MIF	maximal inspiratory flow
MVV	maximal voluntary ventilation
NO	nitric oxide
NSP	nonspecific pattern
P	pressure
Pa_{CO_2}	arterial carbon dioxide tension
PA_{CO_2}	partial pressure of carbon dioxide in the alveoli
Palv	alveolar pressure
Pao	pressure at the mouth
Pa_{O_2}	arterial oxygen tension
PA_{O_2}	partial pressure of oxygen in the alveoli
Patm	atmospheric pressure
P_{CO_2}	partial pressure of carbon dioxide
PEF	peak expiratory flow
PEmax	maximal expiratory pressure
P_{H_2O}	partial pressure of water
PImax	maximal inspiratory pressure
P_{O_2}	partial pressure of oxygen
Ppl	pleural pressure
Pst	lung static elastic recoil pressure
PTLC	lung recoil pressure at TLC
Ptr	pressure inside the trachea
$P\dot{v}_{O_2}$	mixed venous oxygen tension
$\dot{Q}$	perfusion
R	resistance
Raw	airway resistance
Rpulm	pulmonary resistance
RQ	respiratory quotient

RV	residual volume
SAD	small airway disease
SBD$_{LCO}$	single-breath method for estimating D$_{LCO}$
SBN$_2$	single-breath nitrogen (test)
SVC	slow vital capacity
TLC	total lung capacity
V	volume
$\dot{V}$	ventilation
V$_A$	alveolar volume
$\dot{V}_A$	alveolar ventilation
VC	vital capacity
$\dot{V}_{CO_2}$	carbon dioxide production
V$_D$	dead space volume
$\dot{V}_E$	ventilation measured at the mouth
$\dot{V}$max	maximal expiratory flow
$\dot{V}_{O_2}$	oxygen consumption
$\dot{V}_{O_2}$max	maximal oxygen consumption
$\dot{V}/\dot{Q}$	ventilation–perfusion
VR	ventilatory reserve
V$_T$	tidal volume

Contents

chapter 1

Introduction

Dr. Hyatt passed away on June 11, 2016, at the age of 91—one of the last of his generation of legendary pulmonary physiologists and the father of the flow–volume curve. He authored many scientific papers covering a wide spectrum of respiratory physiology and pulmonary medicine. He was demanding and perfectionistic in his research but kind and soft-spoken in his personal interactions. He was one of the greats of respiratory physiology and coauthored papers with Jere (Jeremiah) Mead, Sol (Solbert) Permutt, Peter Macklem, Vito Brusasco, Philip Quanjer, Joe (Joseph) Rodarte, and many others. The "Flow Volume Underworld," which they jointly founded as an ideas forum, was memorialized at the 2015 American Thoracic Society meeting. Dr. Hyatt mentored many fellows and was a collaborative coauthor. He remained active in retirement and published many papers as well as this book in his later years. I have attempted to preserve much of his avuncular writing style in this edition of the book, while updating as needed. The current edition was revised with that intent. Chapters 14 and 15 were extensively revised, while other chapters had additions to incorporate new methods and new standards papers, while still maintaining Dr. Hyatt's writing as much as possible. I hope the end result will be a credit to his memory and his many great achievements in the pulmonary function laboratory.

Paul D. Scanlon, MD

Dr. Hyatt's Introduction to the Fourth Edition

Pulmonary function tests can provide important clinical information, yet they are vastly underused. They are designed to identify and quantify defects and abnormalities in the function of the respiratory system and answer questions such as the following: How badly impaired is the patient's lung function? Is airway obstruction present? How severe is it? Does it respond to bronchodilators? Is gas exchange impaired? Is diffusion of oxygen from alveoli to pulmonary capillary blood impaired? Is treatment helping the patient? How great is the surgical risk?

Pulmonary function tests can also answer other clinical questions: Is the patient's dyspnea caused by cardiac or pulmonary dysfunction? Does the patient with chronic cough have occult asthma? Is obesity impairing the patient's pulmonary function? Is the patient's dyspnea caused by weakness of the respiratory muscles?

The tests alone, however, cannot be expected to lead to a clinical diagnosis of, for example, pulmonary fibrosis or emphysema. Test results must be evaluated in light of the history; physical examination; chest radiograph; computed tomography scan, if available; and pertinent laboratory findings. Nevertheless, some test patterns strongly suggest the presence of certain conditions, such as pulmonary fibrosis. In addition, the flow–volume loop associated with lesions of the trachea and upper airway is often so characteristic as to be nearly diagnostic of the presence of such a lesion (see Chapter 2).

As with any procedure, pulmonary function tests have shortcomings. There is some variability in the normal predicted values of various tests. In some studies, this variability is in part caused by mixing asymptomatic smokers with nonsmokers in a "normal" population. Some variability also occurs among laboratories in the ways the tests are performed, the equipment is used, and the results are calculated.

This text assumes that the tests are performed accurately, and it focuses on their clinical significance. This approach is not to downplay the importance of the technician in obtaining accurate data. Procedures such as electrocardiography require relatively little technician training, especially with the new equipment that can detect errors such as faulty lead placement. And, of course, all the patient needs to do is lie still. In marked contrast is the considerable training required before a pulmonary function technician becomes proficient. With spirometry, for example, the patient must be exhorted to put forth maximal effort, and the technician must learn to detect submaximal effort. The patient is a very active participant in several of the tests that are discussed. Many of these tests have been likened to an athletic event—an apt analogy. In our experience, it takes several weeks of intense training before a technician becomes expert in administering common tests such as spirometry. If at all possible, the person interpreting the test results should undergo pulmonary function testing. Experiencing the tests is the best way to appreciate the challenges faced when administering the test to sick, often frightened patients.

However, the main problem with pulmonary function tests is that they are not ordered often enough. Population surveys generally document some abnormality in respiratory function in 5% to 20% of subjects studied. Chronic obstructive pulmonary disease (COPD) is currently the third leading cause of death in the United States. It causes more than 134,000 deaths per year. It is estimated that 16 million people in the United States have COPD. All too often, the condition is not diagnosed until the disease is far advanced. In a significant number of cases, lung disease is still not being detected. If we are to make an impact on COPD, it needs to be detected in the early stage, at which point smoking cessation markedly reduces the likelihood of progression to severe COPD. Figure 1-1 shows the progression of a typical case of COPD. By the time dyspnea occurs, airway obstruction is moderately or severely advanced. Looked at differently, spirometry can detect airway obstruction in COPD 5 to 10 years before dyspnea occurs.

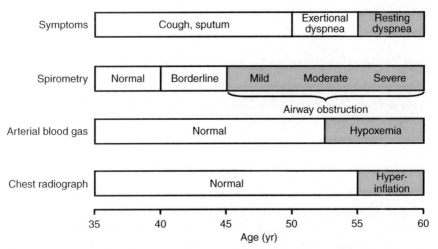

FIG. 1-1 **Typical progression of the symptoms of chronic obstructive pulmonary disease (COPD).** Only spirometry enables the detection of COPD years before shortness of breath develops. (From Enright PL, Hyatt RE, eds. *Office Spirometry: A Practical Guide to the Selection and Use of Spirometers.* Philadelphia, PA: Lea & Febiger, 1987. Used with permission of Mayo Foundation for Medical Education and Research.)

Nevertheless, few primary care physicians routinely order pulmonary function tests for their patients who smoke or for patients with mild-to-moderate dyspnea. For patients with dyspnea, however, in all likelihood, the blood pressure has been checked and chest radiography and electrocardiography have been performed. We have seen patients who have had coronary angiography before simple spirometry identified the true cause of their dyspnea.

Why are so few pulmonary function tests done? It is our impression that a great many clinicians are uncomfortable interpreting the test results. They are not sure what the tests measure or what they mean, and, hence, the tests are not ordered. Unfortunately, very little time is devoted to this subject in medical school and in residency training. Furthermore, it is difficult to determine the practical clinical value of pulmonary function tests from currently available texts of pulmonary physiology and pulmonary function testing. The 2007 Joint Commission Disease-Specific Care Certification Program for the management of COPD (requirement updates go into effect in March 2014) may prompt primary care practitioners to adopt more sensitive and specific diagnostic methods.

The sole purpose of, and justification for, this text is to make pulmonary function tests user friendly. The text targets the basic clinical utility of the most common tests, which also happen to be the most important. Interesting but more complex procedures that have a less important clinical role are left to the standard physiologic texts.

chapter 2

Spirometry: Dynamic Lung Volumes

Spirometry is used to measure the rate at which the lung changes volume during forced breathing maneuvers. The most commonly performed test uses the forced expiratory vital capacity (FVC) maneuver, in which the patient inhales maximally and then exhales as rapidly and completely as possible. Of all the tests considered in this book, the FVC test is both the simplest and the most important. Generally, it provides the most important information obtained from pulmonary function testing. It behooves the reader to have a thorough understanding of this procedure.

2A • Spirograms and Flow–Volume Curve

The two methods of recording the FVC test are shown in Figure 2-1. In Figure 2-1A, the patient blows into a spirometer that records the volume exhaled, which is plotted as a function of time, the solid line. This is the classic spirogram showing the time course of a 4-L FVC. In addition

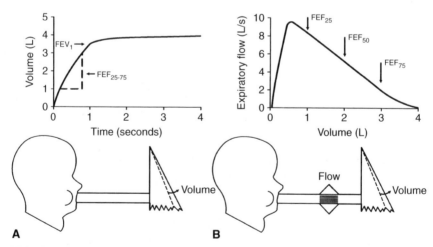

A   **B**

FIG. 2-1 **The two ways to record the forced expiratory vital capacity (FVC) maneuver.** A. Volume recorded as a function of time, the spirogram. FEV_1, forced expiratory volume in 1 second; FEF_{25-75}, average forced expiratory flow rate over the middle 50% of the FVC. B. Flow recorded as a function of volume exhaled, the flow–volume curve. $FEF_{25(50,75)}$, forced expiratory flow after 25% (50%, 75%) of the FVC has been exhaled.

to FVC itself, two of the most common measurements made from this curve are the forced expiratory volume in 1 second (FEV_1) and the average forced expiratory flow (FEF) rate over the middle 50% of the FVC (FEF_{25-75}). These are discussed later in this chapter.

The FVC test can also be plotted as a flow–volume (FV) curve, as in Figure 2-1B. The patient again exhales forcefully into the spirometer through a flowmeter that measures the flow rate (in liters per second) at which the patient exhales. The volume and the rapidity at which the volume is exhaled (flow in liters per second) are plotted as the FV curve. Several of the common measurements made from this curve are discussed later in this chapter.

The two curves reflect the same data, and a computerized spirometer can easily plot both curves, with the patient exhaling through either a flowmeter or a volume recorder. Integration of flow provides volume, which, in turn, can be plotted as a function of time, and all the measurements shown in Figure 2-1 are also readily computed. Conversely, the volume signal can be differentiated with respect to time to determine flow. In our experience, *the FV representation* (Fig. 2-1B) *is the easiest to interpret and the most informative.* Therefore, we will use this representation almost exclusively.

Historical Note: Dr. Hyatt, with Dr. Donald Fry, first described the expiratory flow–volume curve in their classic paper in 1960.[1]

Caution: It is extremely important that the patient be instructed and coached to perform the test properly. Expiration must be after a maximal inhalation, initiated as rapidly as possible and continued with maximal effort until no more air can be expelled. "Good" and "bad" efforts are shown later on page 14 in Figure 2-6.

2B • Value of the Forced Expiratory Vital Capacity Test

The FVC test is the most important pulmonary function test for the following reason: For any given individual during expiration, there is a unique limit to the maximal flow that can be reached at any lung volume. This limit is reached with moderate expiratory efforts, and increasing the force used during expiration does not increase the flow. In Figure 2-1B, consider the maximal FV curve obtained from a normal subject during the FVC test. Once peak flow has been achieved, the rest of the curve defines the maximal flow that can be achieved at any lung volume. Thus, at FEF after 50% of the vital capacity has been exhaled (FEF_{50}), the patient cannot exceed a flow of 5.2 L/s regardless of how hard he or she tries. Note that the maximal flow that can be achieved decreases in an orderly fashion as more air is exhaled (i.e., as lung volume decreases) until at residual volume (4 L) no more air can be exhaled. The FVC test is powerful because there is a limit to maximal expiratory flow at all lung volumes after the first 10% to 15% of FVC has been exhaled. Each individual has a unique maximal expiratory FV curve. Because this curve defines a limit to flow, the curve is highly reproducible in a given patient. Most important, maximal flow is very sensitive to the most common diseases that affect the lung.

The basic physics and aerodynamics causing this flow-limiting behavior are not explained here. However, the concepts are illustrated in the simple lung model in Figure 2-2.

Figure 2-2A shows the lung at full inflation before a forced expiration. Figure 2-2B shows the lung during a forced expiration. As volume decreases, dynamic compression of the airway produces a critical narrowing that develops in the trachea and produces limitation of flow. As expiration continues and lung volume decreases even more, the narrowing migrates distally into the main bronchi and beyond. Three features of the model determine the maximal expiratory flow of the lung at any given lung volume: *lung elasticity* (e), which drives the flow and holds the airways open; *size* of the airways (f); and *resistance* to flow along these airways.

The great value of the FVC test is that it is very sensitive to diseases that alter the lung's mechanical properties:

1. In chronic obstructive pulmonary disease, emphysema causes a loss of lung tissue (alveoli are destroyed). This loss results in a

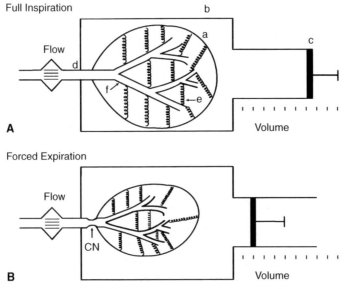

FIG. 2-2 Simple lung model at full inflation (A) and during a forced expiration (B). The lung (a) is contained in a thorax (b) whose volume can be changed by the piston (c). Air exits from the lung via the trachea (d). The lung has elasticity (e), which both drives the flow and plays a role in holding the compliant bronchi (f) open. Critical narrowing (CN) occurs during the forced expiratory vital capacity maneuver.

loss of elastic recoil pressure, which is the driving pressure for maximal expiratory flow. Airways are narrowed because of loss of tethering of lung tissue. This results in increased flow resistance and decreased maximal expiratory flow.

2. In chronic bronchitis, both mucosal thickening and thick secretions in the airways lead to airway narrowing, increased resistance to flow, and decreased maximal flow.

3. In asthma, the airways are narrowed as a result of bronchoconstriction and mucosal inflammation and edema. This narrowing increases resistance and decreases maximal flow.

4. In pulmonary fibrosis, the increased tissue elasticity may distend the airways and increase maximal flow, even though lung volume is reduced.

2C • Reference or Normal Values

Tables and equations are used to determine the normal or predicted values of the measurements to be discussed. The reference values have been derived from large groups of nonsmoking, normal subjects. The important prediction variables are the height, sex, and age of the subject. Certain races, African American and Asian, for example, require race-specific values. These may be obtained from separate race-specific equations or a multiplier applied to the value provided from a single equation. Separate equations are preferred for greater accuracy. Size is best estimated with body height. The taller the subject, the larger the lung and its airways, and thus maximal flows are higher. Women have smaller lungs than men of a given height. With aging, lung elasticity is lost, and thus airways are smaller and flows are lower. The inherent variability in normal predictive values must be kept in mind, however (as in the bell-shaped normal distribution curve of statistics). It is almost never known at what point in the normal distribution a given subject starts. For example, lung disease can develop in people with initially above-average lung volumes and flows. Despite a reduction from their initial baseline, they may still have values within the normal range of a population.

Many different reference equations have been used over the years. Most have been derived from small population samples. The National Health and Nutrition Examination Survey (NHANES or Hankinson) reference equations have been the largest (N = 7,434) and most widely accepted equations in North America until recently. The international Global Lung Function Initiative (GLI) reference values combine the NHANES data with data from many other studies for a total of 57,395 patients. The GLI spirometry reference values are now recommended for most comparisons.

PEARL ● Body height should not be used to estimate normal values for a patient with kyphoscoliosis. Why? Because the decreased height in such a patient will lead to a gross underestimation of the normal lung volume and flows. Instead, the patient's arm span can be measured and used instead of height in the reference equations. In a 40-year-old man with kyphoscoliosis, vital capacity is predicted to be 2.78 L if his height of 147 cm is used, but the correct expected value of 5.18 L is predicted if his arm span of 178 cm is used—a 54% difference. The same principle applies to flow predictions.

2D ● Forced Expiratory Vital Capacity

The FVC is the volume expired during the FVC test; in Figure 2-1 the FVC is 4.0 L. Many abnormalities can cause a decrease in the FVC.

PEARL ● To our knowledge, only one disorder, acromegaly, causes an abnormal *increase* in the FVC. The results of other tests of lung function are usually normal in this condition. However, persons with acromegaly are at increased risk for development of obstructive sleep apnea as a result of hypertrophy of the soft tissues of the upper airway.

Figure 2-3 presents a logical approach to considering possible causes of a decrease in FVC:

1. The problem may be with the *lung* itself. There may have been a resectional surgical procedure or areas of collapse. Various other conditions can render the lung less expandable, such as fibrosis, congestive heart failure, and thickened pleura. Obstructive lung diseases may reduce the FVC by limiting deflation of the lung (Fig. 2-3).

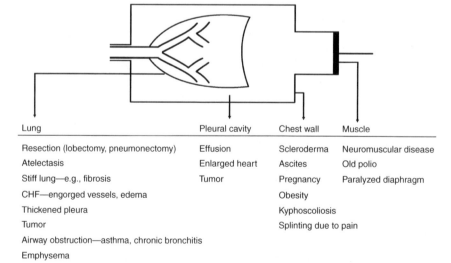

Lung	Pleural cavity	Chest wall	Muscle
Resection (lobectomy, pneumonectomy)	Effusion	Scleroderma	Neuromuscular disease
Atelectasis	Enlarged heart	Ascites	Old polio
Stiff lung—e.g., fibrosis	Tumor	Pregnancy	Paralyzed diaphragm
CHF—engorged vessels, edema		Obesity	
Thickened pleura		Kyphoscoliosis	
Tumor		Splinting due to pain	
Airway obstruction—asthma, chronic bronchitis			
Emphysema			

FIG. 2-3 Various conditions that can restrict the forced expiratory vital capacity. CHF, congestive heart failure.

2. The problem may be in the *pleural cavity*, such as an enlarged heart, pleural fluid, or a tumor encroaching on the lung.
3. Another possibility is restriction of the *chest wall*. The lung cannot inflate and deflate normally if the motion of the chest wall (which includes its abdominal components) is restricted.
4. Inflation and deflation of the system require normal function of the *respiratory muscles*, primarily the diaphragm, the intercostal muscles, and the abdominal muscles.

If the four possibilities listed are considered (lung, pleura, chest wall, and muscles), the cause(s) of decreased FVC is usually determined. Of course, combinations of conditions occur, such as the enlarged failing heart with engorgement of the pulmonary vessels and pleural effusions. It should be remembered that the FVC is a maximally rapid expiratory vital capacity. The vital capacity may be larger when measured at slow flow rates; this situation is discussed in Chapter 3.

Two terms are frequently used in the interpretation of pulmonary function tests. One is an *obstructive defect*. This is a lung disease that causes a decrease in maximal expiratory flow so that rapid emptying of the lungs is not possible; conditions such as emphysema, chronic bronchitis, and asthma cause this. Frequently, an associated decrease in the FVC occurs. A *restrictive defect* implies that lung volume, in this case the total lung capacity (TLC), is reduced by any of the processes listed in Figure 2-3, *except* those causing obstruction.

Caution: In a restrictive process, the TLC will be less than normal (see Chapter 3).

Earlier in the chapter, it was noted that most alterations in lung mechanics lead to decreased maximal expiratory flows. Low expiratory flows resulting from airway obstruction are the hallmark of chronic bronchitis, emphysema, and asthma. The measurements commonly obtained to quantify expiratory obstruction are discussed later.

2E • Forced Expiratory Volume in 1 Second

The FEV_1 is the most reproducible, most commonly obtained, and possibly most useful spirometry measurement. It is the volume of air exhaled in the first second of the FVC test. The normal value depends on the patient's size, age, sex, and race, just as does the FVC. Figure 2-4A and B shows the FVC and FEV_1 from two normal subjects; the larger subject (A) has the larger FVC and FEV_1.

When flow rates are slowed by airway obstruction, as in emphysema, the FEV_1 is decreased by an amount that reflects the severity of the disease. The FVC may also be reduced, although usually to a lesser degree. Figure 2-4C shows a severe degree of obstruction. The FEV_1 is easily

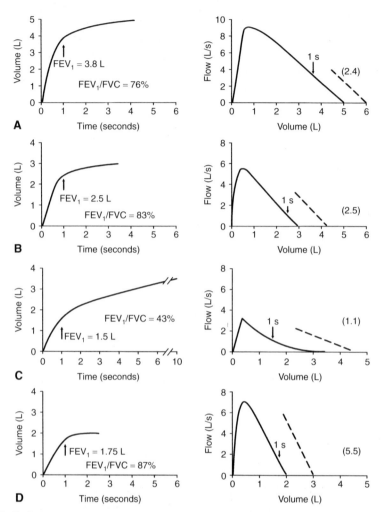

FIG. 2-4 Typical spirograms and flow–volume curves during forced expiration. A and B. Normal patients of different sizes. C. Patient with severe airway obstruction. D. Values typical of a pulmonary restrictive process. The *arrows* indicate the forced expiratory volume in 1 second (FEV_1). The ratios of FEV_1 to forced expiratory vital capacity (FVC) and the slopes of the flow–volume curves (*dashed lines*, values in parentheses) are also shown.

identified directly from the spirogram. A 1-second mark can be added to the FV curve to identify the FEV_1, as shown in the figure. The common conditions producing expiratory slowing or obstruction are chronic bronchitis, emphysema, and asthma.

In Figure 2-4D, the FEV_1 is reduced because of a restrictive defect, such as pulmonary fibrosis. A logical question is "How can I tell whether the FEV_1 is reduced as a result of airway obstruction or a restrictive process?" This question is considered next.

2F • Forced Expiratory Volume in 1 Second/Forced Expiratory Vital Capacity Ratio

The FEV_1/FVC ratio is generally expressed as a percentage. The amount exhaled during the first second is a fairly constant fraction of the FVC, irrespective of lung size. In the normal adult, the ratio ranges from 75% to 85%, but it decreases somewhat with aging. Children have high flows for their size, and thus their ratios are higher, up to 90%.

The significance of this ratio is twofold. First, it aids in quickly identifying persons with airway obstruction in whom the FVC is reduced. For example, in Figure 2-4C, the FEV_1/FVC is very low, at 43%, indicating that the low FVC is likely caused by airway obstruction and not pulmonary restriction. Second, the ratio is valuable for identifying the cause of a low FEV_1. In pulmonary restriction (without any associated obstruction), the FEV_1 and FVC are decreased proportionally; hence, the ratio is in the normal range, as in the case of fibrosis in Figure 2-4D, in which it is 87%. Indeed, in some cases of pulmonary fibrosis, the ratio may increase even more because of the increased elastic recoil of such lungs.

Thus, in regard to the question of how to determine whether airway obstruction or a restrictive process is causing a reduced FEV_1, the answer is to check the FEV_1/FVC ratio. A low FEV_1 with a normal ratio *may* indicate a restrictive process or a nonspecific abnormality (see later in the chapter), whereas a low FEV_1 and a decreased ratio signify a predominantly obstructive process.

In severe obstructive lung disease near the end of a forced expiration, the flows may be very low, barely perceptible. Continuation of the forced expiration can be very tiring and uncomfortable. To avoid patient fatigue, one can substitute the volume expired in 6 seconds, the FEV_6, for the FVC in the ratio. Normal values for FEV_1/FEV_6 were developed in NHANES III.[2]

In 2005,[3] an international group has recommended that the largest vital capacity measured during a study be used in the denominator of the ratio. In most cases, this will be the FVC, but on occasion it will be a slow vital capacity (SVC). When the SVC exceeds the FVC, a patient with a low normal FEV_1/FVC may be moved into the mild obstructive category. The impact and value of this change are yet to be determined (see Chapter 14).

PEARL ● Look at the FV curve. If significant scooping or concavity can be seen, as in Figure 2-4C, obstruction is usually present (older normal adults usually have some degree of scooping). In addition, look at the slope of the FV curve, the average change in flow divided by the change in volume. In normal subjects, this is roughly 2.5 (2.5 L/s per liter). The normal range is approximately 2.0 to 3.0. In the case of airway obstruction (Fig. 2-4C), the average slope is lower, 1.1. In the patient with fibrosis (Fig. 2-4D), the slope is normal to increased, 5.5. The *whole* curve needs to be studied.

Caution: A low FEV_1 and a normal FEV_1/FVC ratio usually indicate restriction with a reduced TLC. However, there is a subset of patients with a low FEV_1, a normal FEV_1/FVC ratio (which rules out obstruction), and a normal TLC (which rules out restriction). We have termed this combination of an abnormally low FEV_1, normal FEV_1/FVC ratio, and normal TLC a "nonspecific pattern" (NSP).[4] (See reference 4 at the end of this chapter and Fig. 3-8.)

2G • Other Measures of Maximal Expiratory Flow

Figure 2-5 shows the other most common measurements of maximal expiratory flow, generally referred to as FEF. All of these measurements are decreased in obstructive disease.

FEF_{25-75} is the average FEF rate over the middle 50% of the FVC. This variable can be measured directly from the spirogram. A microprocessor is used to obtain it from the FV curve. Some clinicians consider the FEF_{25-75} a sensitive indicator of small airways disease or early airway obstruction, but it has a wide range of normal values and is quite nonspecific. Most guidelines now recommend against its use for interpretation of lung function.

FEF_{50} is the flow after 50% of the FVC has been exhaled, and FEF_{75} is the flow after 75% of the FVC has been exhaled. These, too, are no longer recommended for pulmonary function test reports.

Maximal expiratory flow (FEFmax) occurs shortly after the onset of expiration. More than other measures, FEFmax is very dependent on patient effort—the patient must initially exhale as hard as possible to obtain reproducible data. However, with practice, reproducible results are obtainable. The term peak expiratory flow (PEF) is usually applied to the measurement made with a peak flow meter that is not part of a full FVC maneuver. It is similar to FEFmax, but not identical because of the different technique. PEF is usually reported in liters per minute, whereas FEFmax is usually reported in liters per second. Inexpensive portable peak flow measurement devices allow patients to monitor day-to-day variation in PEF at home and so monitor their status. This method is useful mainly for patients with asthma. As shown in Figure 2-5, these other measures, just as with the FEV_1, can be reduced in pure restrictive disease. Again, the FV curve and the FEV_1/FVC ratio must be considered.

2H • How to Estimate Patient Performance from the FV Curve

For most purposes, this book assumes the results of spirometry are accurate. However, it is important that the FVC test be performed correctly, and spirometry interpreters must be able to recognize and comment on suboptimal test performance, which occurs with a small percentage of tests in even the best laboratories. Generally, judgment about the performance

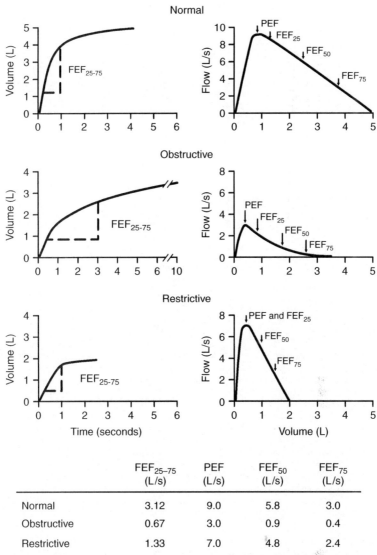

	FEF$_{25-75}$ (L/s)	PEF (L/s)	FEF$_{50}$ (L/s)	FEF$_{75}$ (L/s)
Normal	3.12	9.0	5.8	3.0
Obstructive	0.67	3.0	0.9	0.4
Restrictive	1.33	7.0	4.8	2.4

FIG. 2-5 **Other measurements of maximal expiratory flow in three typical conditions— normal, obstructive disease, and pulmonary restrictive disease.** The average forced expiratory flow (FEF) rate over the middle 50% of the forced expiratory vital capacity (FVC) (FEF$_{25-75}$) is obtained by measuring the volume exhaled over the middle portion of the FVC maneuvers and dividing it by the time required to exhale that volume. FEF$_{25}$, FEF after 25% of the FVC has been exhaled; FEF$_{50}$, flow after 50% of FVC has been exhaled; FEF$_{75}$, flow after 75% of FVC has been exhaled; PEF, peak expiratory flow.

can be made from the FV curve along with technicians' comments. Occasionally, less-than-ideal curves may result from an underlying problem such as muscle weakness.

In Figure 2-6, an excellent effort (A) is contrasted with ones that are unacceptable or require repeating of the test. The three features of the

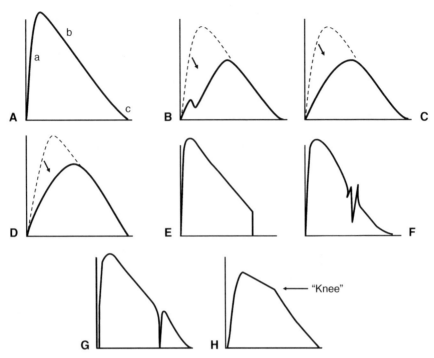

FIG. 2-6 Examples of good and unacceptable forced expiratory vital capacity maneuvers. A. Excellent effort: a, rapid climb to peak flow; b, continuous decrease in flow; c, termination at 0–0.05 L/s of zero flow. B. Hesitating start makes curve unacceptable. C. Patient did not exert maximal effort at start of expiration; test needs to be repeated. D. Such a curve often indicates failure to exert maximal effort initially, but occasionally, it is reproducible and valid. It is sometimes called a *rainbow curve*. It may be found in children, patients with neuromuscular disease, or patients who perform the maneuver poorly. In (B), (C), and (D), the *dashed line* indicates the expected curve; the *arrow* indicates the reduction in flow caused by performance error. E. Curve shows good start, but patient quits too soon; the test needs to be repeated. Occasionally, this is reproducible, and this curve can be normal for some young nonsmokers. F. Coughing during the first second will decrease the forced expiratory volume in 1 second. The maneuver should be repeated. G. Patient stopped exhaling momentarily; test needs to be repeated. H. This curve with a "knee" or "tracheal plateau" is a normal variant that is often seen in nonsmokers, especially young women.

well-performed test are that (1) the curve shows a rapid climb to peak flow (a); (2) the curve then has a fairly smooth, continuous decrease in flow (b); and (3) the curve terminates at a flow within 0.05 L/s of zero flow or, ideally, at zero flow (c). The other curves in Figure 2-6 do not satisfy at least one of these features.

An additional important criterion is that the curves should be repeatable. Ideally, two curves should exhibit the above-described features and have peak flows within 10% of each other and FVC and FEV_1 volumes within 150 mL or 5% of each other. The technician needs to work with the patient to satisfy these repeatability criteria. The physician must examine the selected curve for the contour characteristics. If the results are not satisfactory, the test may be repeated so that the data truly reflect the mechanical properties of a patient's lungs. A suboptimal test must be interpreted with caution because it may suggest the presence of disease when none exists.

2I • Maximal Voluntary Ventilation

The test for maximal voluntary ventilation (MVV) is an athletic event. The patient is instructed to breathe as *hard* and *fast* as possible for 10 to 15 seconds. The best 6 to 12 seconds is measured, and the result is extrapolated to 60 seconds and reported in liters per minute. There can be a significant learning effect with this test, but a skilled technician can coach the patient to avoid problems.

A low MVV relative to FEV_1 suggests variable extrathoracic (upper airway) obstruction, respiratory muscular weakness, or poor test performance. The test is nonspecific but does correlate with a patient's exercise capacity and with the complaint of dyspnea. It is considered useful for estimating a patient's ability to withstand certain types of operations (see Chapter 10).

PEARL ● A normal MVV is approximately equal to the $FEV_1 \times 40$. If the FEV_1 is 3.0 L, the MVV should be approximately 120 L/min (40×3). On the basis of a review of many pulmonary function tests, we set the lower limit of the predicted MVV at $FEV_1 \times 30$. Example: A patient's FEV_1 is 2.5 L and the MVV is 65 L/min. The $FEV_1 \times 30$ is 75 L/min, and thus the MVV of 65 L/min may lead to a suspicion of poor test performance or fatigue. There are two important pathologic causes for the MVV to be less than the predicted lower limit in an otherwise normal subject: obstructing lesions of the major airways (see Section 2K, page 16) and respiratory muscle weakness (see Section 9D, page 86). An MVV much greater than $FEV_1 \times 40$ may mean that the FEV_1 test was poorly performed. However, this product estimate may be less useful in advanced obstructive disease, when the patient's MVV sometimes exceeds that predicted from the FEV_1 (see Chapter 15, case 20, page 173).

PEARL ● Some lesions of the major airway (see page 18, the Pearl) cause the MVV to be reduced out of proportion to the FEV_1. The same result can occur in patients who have muscle weakness, as in neuromuscular diseases (amyotrophic lateral sclerosis, myasthenia gravis, and polymyositis). Thus, these conditions need to be considered when the MVV is reduced out of proportion to the FEV_1.

2J • Maximal Inspiratory Flows

All modern spirometry systems allow measurement of both expiratory and inspiratory flows. The usual approach to measuring inspiratory flows is shown in Figure 2-7A. The patient exhales maximally (the FVC test) and then immediately inhales as rapidly

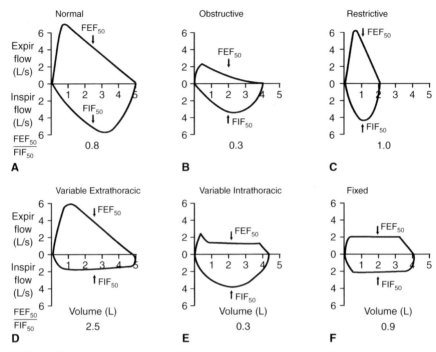

FIG. 2-7 Comparison of typical flow–volume loops (A–C) with the classic flow–volume loops in cases of lesions of the major airway (D–F). Inspiratory flow should always exceed expiratory flow at that volume. If not, an upper airway (extrathoracic) obstruction should be considered. FEF_{50}, forced expiratory flow (expir flow) after 50% of the FVC has been exhaled; FIF_{50}, forced inspiratory flow (inspir flow) measured at the same volume as FEF_{50}.

and completely as possible, producing an inspiratory curve. The combined expiratory and inspiratory FV curves form the *FV loop*. Increased airway resistance decreases both maximal expiratory flow and maximal inspiratory flow (MIF). However, unlike expiration, in which there is a limit to maximal flow, no mechanism such as dynamic compression limits MIF. Thus, it is very effort dependent.

The use of measurement of inspiratory flows is highly variable between laboratories. Some laboratories perform them routinely for all patients, an unnecessary expense in our opinion. Others rarely obtain them, perhaps missing important pathology. The main value of testing MIF is for detecting lesions of the major airways.

2K • Obstructing Lesions of the Major Airway

Obstructing lesions involving the central airway (carina to oropharynx) are relatively uncommon. When present, however, they can often be detected by changes in the FV loop.[5] This is a very important diagnosis to make.

The identification of these lesions from the FV loop depends on two characteristics. One is the *behavior* of the lesion during rapid expiration and inspiration. Does the lesion narrow and decrease flow excessively during one or the other of the phases of respiration? If it does, the lesion is categorized as *variable*. If the lesion is narrowed and decreases flow equally during both phases, the lesion is categorized as *fixed*. The other characteristic is the *location* of the lesion. Is it *extrathoracic* (above the thoracic outlet) or *intrathoracic* (to and including the carina but generally not beyond)?

Figure 2-7 illustrates typical FV loops in normal subjects (Fig. 2-7A), various disease states (Fig. 2-7B and C), and the three classic loops caused by lesions of the major airway (Fig. 2-7D–F). The factors that determine the unique contours of the curves for lesions of the major airway can be appreciated by considering the relationship between the intra-airway and extra-airway pressures during these forced maneuvers.

During *forced expiration*, the airway pressure in the intrathoracic trachea (Ptr) is less than the surrounding pleural pressure (Ppl), and this airway region normally narrows. The airway pressure in the extrathoracic trachea (Ptr) is higher than the surrounding atmospheric pressure (Patm), and the region tends to stay distended. During *forced inspiration*, Ptr in the extrathoracic portion is lower than the surrounding pressure (i.e., Patm), and therefore this region tends to narrow. In the intrathoracic trachea, the surrounding Ppl is more negative than Ptr, which favors dilatation of this region. In the *variable* lesions, these normal changes in airway size are greatly exaggerated.

Figure 2-7D shows results with a *variable* lesion in the *extrathoracic* trachea. This may be caused by, for example, paralyzed but mobile vocal cords. This is explained by the model in Figure 2-8 (left). During expiration, the high intra-airway pressure (Ptr) keeps the cords distended, and there may be little effect on expiratory flow. Ptr is greater than Patm

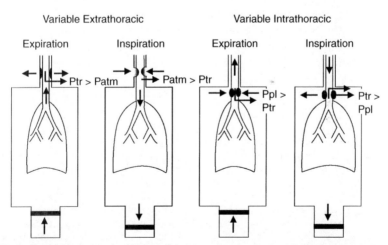

FIG. 2-8 Model explaining the pathophysiology of the variable lesion of the major airway. Patm, atmospheric pressure acting on the extrathoracic trachea; Ppl, pressure in the pleural cavity that acts on the intrathoracic trachea; Ptr, lateral, intratracheal airway pressure.

acting on the outside of this lesion. During inspiration, however, the low pressure in the trachea causes marked narrowing of the cords with the remarkable reduction in flow seen in the inspiratory FV loop because Patm now greatly exceeds airway pressure, Ptr.

The model in Figure 2-8 (right) also explains Figure 2-7E, a *variable intrathoracic* lesion, for example, a compressible tracheal malignancy. During forced expiration, the high Ppl relative to Ptr produces a marked narrowing with a dramatic constant reduction in expiratory flow in the FV loop. Yet inspiratory flow may be little affected because Ppl is more negative than airway pressure, and the lesion distends.

Figure 2-7F shows the characteristic loop with *a fixed*, orifice-like lesion. Such a lesion—for example, a napkin-ring cancer of the trachea or fixed, narrowed, paralyzed vocal cords—interferes almost equally with expiratory and inspiratory flows. The location of the lesion does not matter because the lesion does not change size regardless of the intra-airway and extra-airway pressures.

Various indices have been used to characterize these lesions of the major airway. Figure 2-7 shows the ratio of expiratory to inspiratory flow at 50% of the vital capacity (FEF_{50}/FIF_{50}). The ratio deviates most dramatically from the other curves in the variable lesion in the extrathoracic trachea (Fig. 2-7D). The ratio is nonspecific in the other lesions. The unique FV loop contours of the various lesions are the principal diagnostic features. Once a lesion of the major airway is suspected, confirmation by direct endoscopic visualization or radiographic imaging of the lesion is required.

Caution: Because some lesions may be predominantly, but not absolutely, variable or fixed, intermediate patterns can occur, but the loops are usually sufficiently abnormal to raise suspicion.

The spirograms corresponding to the lesions in Figure 2-7D through F are not shown because they are not nearly as useful as the FV loops for detecting these lesions. Some of the clinical situations in which we have encountered these abnormal FV loops are listed in Table 2-1.

PEARL ● If an isolated, significant *decrease* in the MVV occurs in association with a normal FVC, FEV_1, and FEF_{25-75}, or if the MVV is reduced well out of proportion to the reduction in the FEV_1, a major airway obstruction should be strongly suspected. A forced inspiratory vital capacity loop needs to be obtained. Of course, an inspiratory loop is also mandated if there is a plateau on the expiratory curve (Fig. 2-7E and F). Not all laboratories routinely measure inspiratory loops. The technician needs to be asked whether stridor was heard during the MVV—it often is. In most such cases at our institution, these lesions are identified by technicians who find an unexplained low MVV or may hear stridor. They then obtain the inspiratory loop, which can lead to an important diagnosis. Another consideration is whether the patient has a neuromuscular disorder, as discussed in Section 9D.

> **PEARL** ● If your laboratory does not routinely provide a maximal inspiratory FV loop, you should order one if your patient has any of the following: (1) inspiratory stridor; (2) isolated reduction in the MVV; (3) significant dyspnea with no apparent cause and with normal spirometry; (4) atypical asthma; or (5) a history of thyroid surgery, prolonged intubation or tracheotomy, vocal cord dysfunction, goiter, or neck radiation.

2L • Small Airway Disease

Small airway disease, that is, disease of the peripheral airways, is an established pathologic finding. However, it has been difficult to develop tests that are specific indicators of small airway dysfunction. Tests such as density dependence of maximal expiratory flow and frequency dependence of compliance are difficult to perform and relatively nonspecific. (They are not discussed here.) Chapter 8 discusses the closing volume and the slope of phase III. The slope of phase III is very sensitive but relatively nonspecific. The data that may best reflect peripheral airway function are the flows measured at low lung volumes during the FVC tests. These include the FEF_{25-75}, FEF_{50}, and FEF_{75} (see Fig. 2-5, page 13), but these tests have such a wide range of variation of normal values that they are no longer recommended for interpretation of lung function.

TABLE 2-1 Examples of Lesions of the Major Airway Detected with the Flow–Volume Loop

Variable extrathoracic lesions

Vocal cord paralysis (due to thyroid operation, tumor invading recurrent laryngeal nerve, amyotrophic lateral sclerosis, post-polio)

Subglottic stenosis

Neoplasm (primary hypopharyngeal or tracheal, metastatic from primary lesion in lung or breast)

Goiter

Variable intrathoracic lesions

Tumor of lower trachea (below sternal notch)

Tracheomalacia

Strictures

Granulomatosis with polyangiitis (formerly called Wegener granulomatosis) or relapsing polychondritis

Fixed lesions

Fixed neoplasm in central airway (at any level)

Vocal cord paralysis with fixed stenosis

Fibrotic stricture

2M • Typical Spirometric Patterns

The typical test patterns discussed are summarized in Table 2-2. Because test results are nonspecific in lesions of the major airway, they are not included, the most diagnostically useful measure being the contour of the full FV loop.

2N • Gestalt Approach to Interpretation

Rather than merely memorizing patterns such as those listed in Table 2-2, another approach that is very useful is to visually compare the individual FV curve with the normal predicted curve (see Chapter 14).

In Figure 2-9A, the dashed curve is the patient's normal, predicted FV curve. As a first approximation, this curve can be viewed as defining the maximal expiratory flows and volumes that can be achieved by the patient. In other words, it defines a mechanical limit to ventilation, and all expiratory flows are usually on or beneath the curve (i.e., within the *area* under the curve).

Assume that chronic obstructive pulmonary disease develops in the patient with the normal, predicted curve in Figure 2-9A, and then the curve becomes that shown in Figure 2-9B. At a glance, this plot provides a lot of information. First, the patient has lost a great deal of the normal area (the shaded area) and is confined to breathing in the reduced area

TABLE 2-2 **Typical Patterns of Impairment**		
Measurement	**Obstructive**	**Restrictive**
FVC (L)	N to ↓	↓
FEV_1 (L)	↓	↓
FEV_1/FVC (%)	N to ↓	N to ↑
FEF_{25-75} (L/s)	↓	N to ↓
PEF (L/s)	N to ↓	N to ↓
FEF_{50} (L/s)	↓	N to ↓
Slope of FV curve	↓	↑
MVV (L/min)	↓	N to ↓

FEF_{25-75}, forced expiratory flow rate over the middle 50% of the FVC; FEF_{50}, forced expiratory flow after 50% of the FVC has been exhaled; FEV_1, forced expiratory volume in 1 second; FV, flow–volume; FVC, forced expiratory vital capacity; MVV, maximal voluntary ventilation; N, normal; PEF, peak expiratory flow; ↓, decreased; ↑, increased.

Comments:
1. If pulmonary fibrosis is suspected as the cause of restriction, diffusing capacity (see Chapter 4) and total lung capacity (see Chapter 3) should be determined.
2. If muscle weakness is suspected as a cause of restriction, maximal respiratory pressures should be determined (see Chapter 9).
3. For assessing the degree of emphysema, total lung capacity and diffusing capacity (see Chapters 3 and 4) should be determined.
4. If asthma is suspected, testing should be repeated after bronchodilator therapy (see Chapter 5).

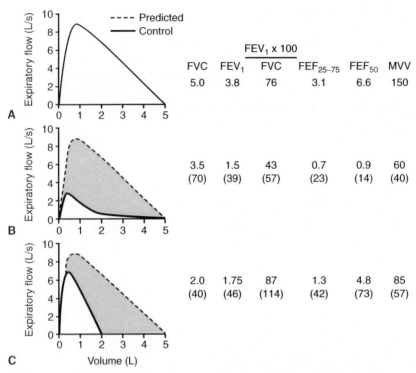

	FVC	FEV$_1$	$\dfrac{FEV_1 \times 100}{FVC}$	FEF$_{25-75}$	FEF$_{50}$	MVV
A	5.0	3.8	76	3.1	6.6	150
B	3.5	1.5	43	0.7	0.9	60
	(70)	(39)	(57)	(23)	(14)	(40)
C	2.0	1.75	87	1.3	4.8	85
	(40)	(46)	(114)	(42)	(73)	(57)

FIG. 2-9 **The gestalt approach to interpreting pulmonary function data when the predicted and observed flow–volume curves are available.** The shaded area between the predicted and measured curves (B and C) provides a visual index of the degree of ventilatory limitation, there being none for the normal subject in (A). (B) is typical of severe airway obstruction. (C) is typical of a severe pulmonary restrictive process. FEF$_{25-75}$, forced expiratory flow rate over the middle 50% of the FVC; FEF$_{50}$, forced expiratory flow after 50% of the FVC has been exhaled; FEV$_1$, forced expiratory volume in 1 second; FVC, forced vital capacity; MVV, maximal voluntary ventilation.

under the measured curve. Clearly, severe ventilatory limitation is present. The concave shape of the FV curve and the low slope indicate an *obstructive* process. Before one even looks at the values to the right, it can be determined that the FVC and PEF are reduced and that the FEV$_1$, FEV$_1$/FVC ratio, FEF$_{25-75}$, and FEF$_{50}$ must also be reduced. Because the MVV is confined to this reduced area, it too will be decreased. The numbers in the figure confirm this.

Next, consider Figure 2-9C, in which the patient has interstitial pulmonary fibrosis. Again, a glance at the plot reveals a substantial loss of area, indicating a moderately severe ventilatory limitation. The steep slope of the FV curve and the reduced FVC are consistent with the process being *restrictive*. A reduced FEV$_1$ but a normal FEV$_1$/FVC ratio can also be determined, and the flow rates (FEF$_{25-75}$ and FEF$_{50}$) can be expected to be normal to reduced. The MVV will be better preserved than that shown in Figure 2-9B because high expiratory flows can still develop, albeit over a restricted volume range. The numbers confirm these conclusions.

The gestalt approach can be a useful first step in analyzing pulmonary function data. Dr. Hyatt estimated the degree of ventilatory limitation on the basis of loss of area under the normal predicted FV curve, the shaded areas in Figure 2-9B and C. He arbitrarily defined an area loss of 25% as mild, 50% as moderate, and 75% as severe ventilatory limitation, although that does not necessarily correlate with other systems for grading the severity of impairment on pulmonary function tests.

REFERENCES

1. Fry DL, Hyatt RE. Pulmonary mechanics. *Am J Med* 29:672, 1960.
2. Hankinson JL, Odencrantz JR, Fedan KB. Spirometric reference values from a sample of the general U.S. population. *Am J Respir Crit Care Med* 159:179–187, 1999.
3. Pellegrino R, Viegi G, Brusasco V, et al. Interpretative strategies for lung function tests. *Eur Respir J* 26:948–968, 2005.
4. Hyatt RE, Cowl CT, Bjoraker JA, Scanlon PD. Conditions associated with an abnormal non-specific pattern of pulmonary function tests. *Chest* 135:419–424, 2009.
5. Miller RD, Hyatt RE. Obstructing lesions of the larynx and trachea: clinical and physiologic characteristics. *Mayo Clin Proc* 44:145–161, 1969.

chapter 3

Static (Absolute) Lung Volumes

Measures of the so-called static (or absolute) lung volumes are often informative.[1] The most important are the vital capacity (VC), residual volume (RV), and total lung capacity (TLC). The VC is measured by having the patient inhale maximally and then exhale *slowly* and completely. This VC is called the *slow vital capacity* (SVC). Similar to the SVC is the inspiratory vital capacity (IVC). The patient breathes normally and then exhales slowly and completely and inhales maximally. The SVC and the IVC provide similar results. The SVC is used in this book rather than the IVC.

With complete exhaling, air still remains in the lung. This remaining volume is the RV. The RV can be visualized by comparing the inspiratory and expiratory chest radiographs (Fig. 3-1). The fact that the lungs do not collapse completely on full expiration is important physiologically. With complete collapse, transient hypoxemia would occur because mixed venous blood reaching the lung would have no oxygen to pick up. Furthermore, inflation of a collapsed lung requires very high inflating pressures, which would quickly fatigue the respiratory muscles and could tear the lung, leading to a *pneumothorax*. This is the problem in infants born with respiratory distress syndrome, in which portions of the lung can collapse (individual acinar units, up to whole lobes) at the end of exhalation.

The RV can be measured and added to the SVC to obtain the TLC. Alternatively, the TLC can be measured and the SVC subtracted from it to obtain the RV. The value of these volumes is discussed below.

3A • Slow Vital Capacity

Normally, the SVC and forced expiratory vital capacity (FVC; discussed in Chapter 2) are identical, as shown in the top panel of Figure 3-2. With airway obstruction, as in chronic obstructive pulmonary disease (COPD) or asthma, the FVC can be considerably smaller than the SVC, as shown in the lower panel of Figure 3-2. The difference between SVC and FVC reflects trapping of air in the lungs. The higher flows during the FVC maneuver cause excessive narrowing and closure of diseased airways in COPD, and thus the lung cannot empty as completely as during the SVC maneuver. Although trapping is of interest to the physiologist, it is of limited value as a clinical measure. However, it does explain the possible discrepancies between the volumes of the SVC and the FVC.

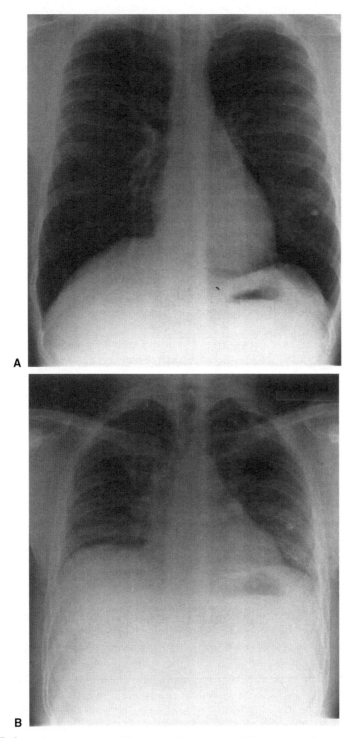

FIG. 3-1 Radiographs obtained from a healthy patient at full inspiration (i.e., at total lung capacity, A) and full expiration (B), in which the air remaining in the lung is the residual volume.

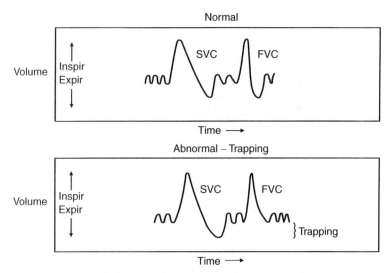

FIG. 3-2 Spirogram for a normal patient during various maneuvers compared with that of a patient with obstructive lung disease who shows trapping. Expir, expiration; FVC, forced expiratory vital capacity; Inspir, inspiration; SVC, slow vital capacity.

3B • Residual Volume and Total Lung Capacity

Figure 3-3 depicts the static lung volumes that are of most interest. The RV is measured (see page 26) and added to the SVC to obtain the TLC. The *expiratory reserve volume* (ERV) is the volume of air that can be exhaled after a normal expiration during quiet breathing (tidal breathing). The volume used during tidal breathing is the *tidal volume*. The *inspiratory reserve volume* is the volume of air that can be inhaled at the end

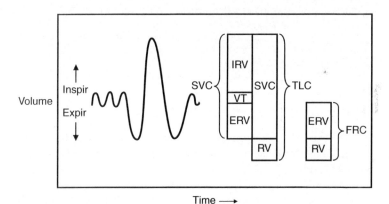

FIG. 3-3 Various static (or absolute) lung volumes. Total lung capacity (TLC) is the sum of the residual volume (RV) and slow vital capacity (SVC). The SVC is the sum of the inspiratory reserve volume (IRV), the tidal volume (VT), and the expiratory reserve volume (ERV). The functional residual capacity (FRC) is the sum of the RV and the ERV. Expir, expiration; Inspir, inspiration.

of a normal tidal inspiration. The sum of the ERV and RV is termed the *functional residual capacity* (FRC).

RV is the remaining volume of air in the lung at the end of a complete expiratory maneuver. It is determined by the limits of either the chest wall excursion or airway collapse or compression. In restrictive disorders, the limit of chest wall compression by the chest wall muscles determines RV. In obstructive disorders, the collapse of airways prevents air escape from the lungs, thereby determining the maximal amount exhaled. In obstructive disease, the RV is increased. There is one exception. The RV can be increased in a few young, healthy adults who are unable to completely compress their chest wall. In these cases, a curve like the one shown in Figure 2-6E is produced. The TLC is increased in most patients with chronic obstruction. However, TLC is often not increased in asthma. Finally, for a confident diagnosis of a *restrictive* process, the TLC must be *decreased.*

The FRC is primarily of interest to the physiologist. It is the lung volume at which the inward elastic recoil of the lung is balanced by the outward elastic forces of the relaxed chest wall (rib cage and abdomen). It is normally 40% to 50% of the TLC. When lung elasticity is reduced, as in emphysema, the FRC increases. It also increases to a lesser extent with normal aging. With the increased lung recoil in pulmonary fibrosis, the FRC decreases.

PEARL ● The FRC is normally less when a patient is supine than when sitting or standing. When a person is upright, the heavy abdominal contents pull the relaxed diaphragm down, expanding both the rib cage and the lungs. In the supine position, gravity no longer pulls the abdominal contents downward; instead, the contents tend to push the diaphragm up, and thus the FRC is decreased. The lower FRC and, hence, smaller lung volume in the supine position may interfere with gas exchange in patients with various types of lung disease and in the elderly. Blood drawn while these patients are supine may show an abnormally low tension of oxygen in arterial blood. A similar effect often occurs in very obese patients.

3C • How Lung Volumes Are Measured

Usually, the FRC is measured by one of the methods to be described. If the ERV is subtracted from the FRC, the RV is obtained, and, as noted previously, if the RV is added to the SVC, the TLC is obtained (Fig. 3-3).

As shown in Figure 3-2, the SVC may be larger than the FVC in obstructive disease. If the FVC is added to the RV, the TLC will be smaller than if the SVC is used. Conversely, if the FVC is less than the SVC and the RV is calculated by subtracting the FVC from the measured TLC, you will calculate an RV that is high. By convention, and in this book, the SVC is used to compute static lung volume. Alternatively, in the United

States, the FVC, not the SVC, is used to compute the FEV_1/FVC ratio (ratio of the forced expiratory volume in 1 second to the FVC). European reference equations use FEV_1/SVC, also called the Tiffeneau index.

The three most commonly used methods of measuring the FRC (from which the RV is obtained) are nitrogen washout, inert gas dilution, and plethysmography. If these are not available, a radiographic method can be used.

Nitrogen Washout Method

The principle of this procedure is illustrated in Figure 3-4. At the end of a normal expiration, the patient is connected to the system.

The lung contains an unknown volume (Vx) of air containing 75% to 78% nitrogen. With inspiration of nitrogen-free oxygen and exhalation into a separate bag, all the nitrogen can be washed out of the lung. The volume of the expired bag and its nitrogen concentration are measured, and the unknown volume is obtained with the simple mass balance equation. In practice, the procedure is terminated after 7 minutes and not all the nitrogen is removed from the lung, but this is easily corrected for. This procedure underestimates the FRC in patients with airway obstruction because in this condition there are lung regions that are very poorly ventilated, and hence they lose very little of their nitrogen. A truer estimate in obstructive disease can be obtained if this test is prolonged to 15 to 20 minutes. However, patients then find the test unpleasant.

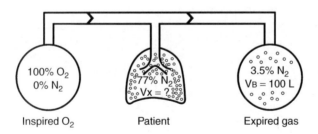

Inspired O_2 Patient   Expired gas

Initial volume of N_2 in patient = 0.8 (Vx)
Vx = FRC
Final volume of N_2 in expired bag = 0.035 (VB)
VB = volume of bag = 0.035 (100)
There is no loss of N_2 from system
so initial N_2 volume = final N_2 volume
0.8 (Vx) = (0.035)(100)
Vx = 4.37 L = FRC

FIG. 3-4 Nitrogen washout method of measuring the functional residual capacity (FRC). The initial volume of nitrogen (N_2) in the lungs at FRC equals 77% N_2 × FRC volume. The N_2 volume of the inhaled oxygen (O_2) is zero. The volume of N_2 washed out of the lung is computed as shown, and the FRC, or Vx, is obtained by solving the mass balance equation, 0.77 (Vx) = 0.035 (VB).

Inert Gas Dilution Technique

The concept is illustrated in Figure 3-5. Helium, argon, or neon can be used. The pulmonary function system contains a known volume of gas (V1). (In Fig. 3-5, C_1 is helium with a known concentration.) At FRC, the patient is connected to the system and rebreathes until the helium concentration reaches a plateau, indicating equal concentrations of helium (C_2) in the spirometer and lung. Because essentially no helium is absorbed, Eqs. 1 and 2 can be combined and solved for Vx, the FRC. In practice, oxygen is added to the circuit to replace that consumed by the patient, and carbon dioxide is absorbed to prevent hypercarbia. As with the nitrogen washout technique, the gas dilution method underestimates the FRC in patients with airway obstruction.

Plethysmography

The principle of plethysmography is simple. The theory is based on Boyle's law, which states that the product of the pressure (P) and volume (V) (PV) of a gas is constant under constant temperature (isothermal) conditions. The gas in the lungs is isothermal because of its intimate contact with capillary blood. The technique is shown in Figure 3-6 with the standard constant-volume body plethysmograph. An attractive feature of this technique is that several measurements of RV and TLC can be obtained quickly. This is not possible with the washout and dilution

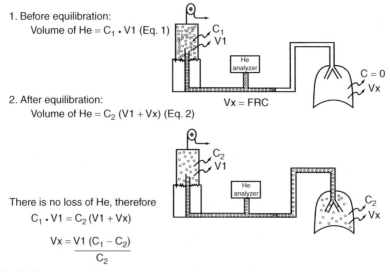

1. Before equilibration:

   Volume of He $= C_1 \cdot V1$ (Eq. 1)

2. After equilibration:

   Volume of He $= C_2 (V1 + Vx)$ (Eq. 2)

   $Vx = FRC$

There is no loss of He, therefore

$$C_1 \cdot V1 = C_2 (V1 + Vx)$$

$$Vx = \frac{V1 (C_1 - C_2)}{C_2}$$

FIG. 3-5 **Helium dilution technique of measuring the functional residual capacity (FRC).** Before the test, no helium (He) is present in the lungs (Vx), and there is a known volume of He in the spirometer and tubing—the concentration of He (C_1) times the volume of the spirometer and the connecting tubes (V1). At equilibrium, the concentration of He (C_2) is uniform throughout the system. The mass balance equation can now be solved for Vx, the FRC.

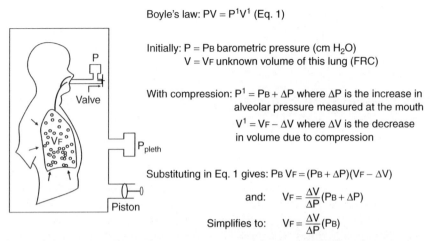

Boyle's law: $PV = P^1V^1$ (Eq. 1)

Initially: $P = P_B$ barometric pressure (cm H_2O)
$V = V_F$ unknown volume of this lung (FRC)

With compression: $P^1 = P_B + \Delta P$ where ΔP is the increase in alveolar pressure measured at the mouth
$V^1 = V_F - \Delta V$ where ΔV is the decrease in volume due to compression

Substituting in Eq. 1 gives: $P_B V_F = (P_B + \Delta P)(V_F - \Delta V)$

and: $V_F = \dfrac{\Delta V}{\Delta P}(P_B + \Delta P)$

Simplifies to: $V_F = \dfrac{\Delta V}{\Delta P}(P_B)$

FIG. 3-6 **The equipment and the measurements needed to measure the functional residual capacity (FRC) by using a body plethysmograph and applying Boyle's law (Eq. 1).** The subject is seated in an airtight plethysmograph and the pressure in the plethysmograph (Ppleth) changes with changes in lung volume. When the subject stops breathing, alveolar pressure equals barometric pressure (P_B). Consider what happens if the valve at the mouth is closed at the end of a quiet expiration, that is, at FRC. As the subject makes an expiratory effort against the closed valve, alveolar pressure increases by an amount (ΔP) that is measured by the mouth gauge, P. Lung volume decreases as a result of gas compression, there being no airflow, and hence Ppleth decreases. The change in Ppleth provides a measure of the change in volume (ΔV), as follows. With the subject momentarily not breathing, the piston pump is cycled and the known volume changes produce known changes in Ppleth. These measurements provide all the data needed to solve the above equation for V_F. The final equation is simplified by omitting ΔP from the quantity ($P_B + \Delta P$). Because ΔP is small (~20 cm H_2O) compared with P_B (~1,000 cm H_2O), it can be neglected. PV, product of pressure and volume.

methods because the alveolar gas composition must be brought back to the control state before these tests can be repeated, a process that often takes 10 to 20 minutes in patients with COPD. The plethysmographic method measures essentially all the gas in the lung, including that in poorly ventilated areas. Thus, in COPD, the FRC, RV, and TLC obtained with this method are usually larger and more accurate than those obtained with the gas methods. In some cases, the TLC of a patient with COPD may be 2 to 3 L more with plethysmography than with other methods.

Radiographic Method

If the foregoing methods are not available, radiographic methods can provide a good estimate of TLC. Posterior–anterior and lateral radiographs are obtained while the patient holds his or her breath at TLC. TLC is estimated by either planimetry or the elliptic method.[2] The radiographic technique compares favorably with the body plethysmographic method and is more accurate than the gas methods in patients with COPD. It is also accurate in patients with pulmonary fibrosis. The technique is not difficult but requires that radiographs be obtained at maximal inspiration. Methods have also been developed for calculating TLC from chest computed tomography scans. It can be quite accurate but also depends on obtaining images at TLC.

3D • Significance of RV and TLC

Knowledge of the RV and TLC can help in determining whether a restrictive or an obstructive process is the cause of a decrease in FVC and FEV_1. This distinction is not always apparent from the flow–volume (FV) curves. The chest imaging may help when obvious hyperinflation or fibrosis is present. Interestingly, the presence of emphysema on computed tomogram is not invariably associated with obstruction on pulmonary function testing. In fact, it is one of the common causes of an isolated reduction in diffusing capacity of carbon monoxide (D_{LCO}) with normal spirometry and lung volumes.

As noted in Section 2F, page 11, the FEV_1/FVC ratio usually provides the answer. However, in a patient with asthma who is not wheezing and has a decreased FVC and FEV_1, both the FEV_1/FVC ratio and the slope of the FV curve may be normal. In this case, the RV should be mildly increased, but the TLC is often normal.

The TLC and RV are often increased in COPD, especially emphysema. Usually, the RV is increased proportionately more than the TLC, and thus the RV/TLC ratio is also increased. The TLC and RV are also increased in acromegaly, but the RV/TLC ratio is normal.

By definition, the TLC is reduced in restrictive disease, and the RV may be reduced, but not necessarily. The diagnosis of a restrictive process cannot be made with confidence unless there is evidence of a decreased TLC. The evidence may be the direct measure of TLC or the apparent volume reduction seen on the chest radiograph, or it may be suggested by the presence of a very steep slope of the FV curve (see Fig. 2-4).

PEARL • Lung resection for lung cancer or bronchiectasis decreases the RV and TLC, but this is an unusual restrictive process. Because there is often associated airway obstruction, the RV/TLC may be abnormally high. Furthermore, an obstructive process will be apparent because of the shape of the FV curve and a decreased FEV_1/FVC ratio. This is a mixed restrictive–obstructive pattern.

3E • Expanding the Gestalt Approach to Absolute Lung Volume Data

Figure 3-7 shows the FV curves from Figure 2-9 as a means to consider what changes might be expected in the absolute lung volumes. Figure 3-7A represents findings in a normal subject: TLC of 7 L, RV of 2 L, and RV/TLC ratio of 29%.

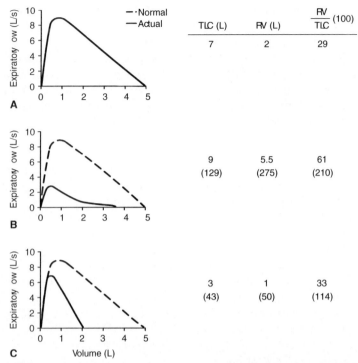

	TLC (L)	RV (L)	$\dfrac{RV}{TLC}$ (100)
A	7	2	29
B	9 (129)	5.5 (275)	61 (210)
C	3 (43)	1 (50)	33 (114)

FIG. 3-7 **Further application of the gestalt approach is introduced in Figure 2-9, page 21.** Note that the area between the predicted (*dashed line*) and observed (*solid line*) flow–volume curves is not shaded. A. Normal pattern, B. Severe obstruction, C. Severe pulmonary restriction. (The numbers in parentheses are the percentages of predicted normal.) RV, residual volume; TLC, total lung capacity.

Figure 3-7B shows a severe ventilatory limitation due to airway obstruction. In addition to the reduced flows, TLC and RV are expected to be increased, RV more than TLC, so that the RV/TLC ratio will also be abnormal. These expectations are confirmed by the values on the right of the figure. However, the effect of lung resection in COPD needs to be considered (see Section 3D).

The FV curve in Figure 3-7C is consistent with severe ventilatory limitation due to a restrictive process. This diagnosis requires the TLC to be decreased, and the RV/TLC ratio is expected to be essentially normal. The values on the right of the figure confirm these expectations.

A question in regard to Figure 3-7C is "What is the cause of this restrictive process?" The answer to this question requires review of Figure 2-3 (page 8), in which all but the obstructive diseases need to be considered. Most restrictive processes can be evaluated from the history, physical examination, and chest radiograph. In fibrosis, diffusing capacity (discussed in Chapter 4) is expected to be reduced and radiographic changes evident. Poor patient effort can usually be *excluded* by evaluating the FV curve (see Fig. 2-6, page 14) and by noting that the patient gives reproducible efforts.

A curve similar to that in Figure 3-7C but with reduced peak flows is found in patients with normal lungs in whom a neuromuscular disorder such as amyotrophic lateral sclerosis develops. In this case, the maximal voluntary ventilation (MVV) is often reduced (see Section 2I, page 15). In addition, with this reduction in the FVC, the maximal respiratory muscle strength is reduced, as discussed in Chapter 9. Interestingly, patients with bilateral diaphragmatic paralysis can present with this pattern. However, these patients differ in that their dyspnea becomes extreme, and often intolerable, when they lie down.

Some massively obese patients also show the pattern in Figure 3-7C. They have a very abnormal ratio of weight (in kilograms) to height^2 (in meters), the body mass index (BMI), which has become the standard index for obesity. A BMI of more than 25 is considered overweight. Anyone with a BMI of 30 or more is considered obese. In our laboratory, we find that a BMI of more than 35 is associated with an average reduction of 5% to 10% in FVC (unpublished data). However, there is a large variation: Some obese individuals have normal lung volumes, and others are more severely affected. These differences are partly related to fat distribution or to the relationship between fat mass and muscle mass.[3] Persons with a large waist measurement or waist/hip ratio are more severely affected.

Figure 3-8 shows two curves in which the FEV_1 and FVC are reduced and the FEV_1/FVC ratio is normal. Both are *consistent* with a restrictive process. However, in both cases the TLC is normal. Therefore, the diagnosis of a restrictive process *cannot* be made. In this case, the term

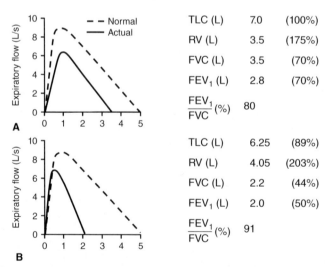

TLC (L)	7.0	(100%)
RV (L)	3.5	(175%)
FVC (L)	3.5	(70%)
FEV_1 (L)	2.8	(70%)
$\dfrac{FEV_1}{FVC}$ (%)	80	

TLC (L)	6.25	(89%)
RV (L)	4.05	(203%)
FVC (L)	2.2	(44%)
FEV_1 (L)	2.0	(50%)
$\dfrac{FEV_1}{FVC}$ (%)	91	

FIG. 3-8 A and B. Examples of nonspecific pattern in which the forced expiratory volume in 1 second (FEV_1) and forced expiratory vital capacity (FVC) are reduced proportionately, giving a normal FEV_1/FVC ratio, and the total lung capacity (TLC) is normal. The numbers in parentheses are the percentages of predicted normal. Note that the residual volume (RV) is increased. This should not be confused with the previously discussed obstructive disorders in which RV is also increased. See Section 3G.

nonspecific pattern (NSP) is applied (see Section 2F, pages 11 and 12, and Section 3G, page 12).

Sometimes a more definitive diagnosis can be made. For example, Figure 3-8A shows a parallel shift of the FV curve. Ventilatory limitation is mild to moderate. This finding is common in mild asthma.[4] The TLC is normal, and the RV and RV/TLC are mildly increased. The history may be consistent with asthma with or without wheezing. The patient often has a higher than normal increase in expiratory flows on the FV curve after use of an inhaled bronchodilator. If this does not occur, a methacholine challenge or exhaled nitric oxide measurement may be recommended in an attempt to uncover a possible asthmatic process. These procedures are discussed in Chapter 5.

Figure 3-8B is an NSP of moderate degree. In this case, the slope of the FV curve is increased, but there is no clinical evidence of parenchymal involvement, and the pulmonary diffusing capacity (D_{LCO}, see Chapter 4) is normal, as is the TLC. This pattern can also occur in patients with relatively quiescent asthma. A thorough history and physical examination may uncover the problem. The response to a bronchodilator may be marked, or the results of the methacholine challenge test may be positive.

We studied a random sample of 100 patients with NSP (reference 4, Chapter 2). All had a TLC by plethysmography and a diffusing capacity within normal limits; thus, restriction was ruled out. There were 62 men and 38 women 20 years old or older. Airway hyperreactivity based on bronchodilator response or methacholine challenge was common. Fifty of the patients were obese. Evidence of COPD was present in 16% despite a normal FEV_1/FVC ratio. If this NSP is found, testing for airway hyperreactivity should be done by either the bronchodilator or the methacholine method, and occasionally both may be indicated. In a later study of 1,289 patients, the NSP persisted in 64% of the patients for at least 3 years.[5] Normal predicted values of the FV curves are relied on heavily. Table 3-1 is an expansion of Table 2-2 (page 20): the TLC, RV, and RV/TLC ratio are added.

3F • Mixed Obstructive–Restrictive Pattern

Occasionally, you may encounter a patient with no history of lung resection whose test shows a reduced TLC (restriction) as well as a reduced FEV_1/FVC ratio (obstruction). This occurs in 1% to 2% of complete pulmonary function tests. To assess the degree of obstruction, you usually use the percent reduction in the FEV_1. However, in this case, some of the reduction in FEV_1 is due to the reduced TLC. To correct for this, the following approach is recommended[6]: Divide the measured FEV_1 percent predicted by the measured TLC percent predicted. For example, a subject has a TLC of 6 L which is 70% predicted and a FEV_1 of 40% predicted. The 40% FEV_1 is divided by the 70% TLC (40/70 = 57% predicted). So the degree of obstruction is adjusted up from 40% to 57%, a moderate or moderately severe degree, rather than a severe degree.

TABLE 3-1 **Typical Patterns of Impairment**

Measurement	Obstructive	Restrictive
FVC (L)	↓	↓
FEV$_1$ (L)	↓	↓
FEV$_1$/FVC (%)	N to ↓	N to ↑
FEF$_{25-75}$ (L/s)	↓	N to ↓
PEF (L/s)	N to ↓	N to ↓
FEF$_{50}$ (L/s)	↓	N to ↓
Slope of FV curve	↓	↑
MVV (L/min)	↓	N to ↓
TLC	N to ↑	↓
RV	↑	↓ to N to ↑
RV/TLC (%)	↑	N to ↑

FEF$_{25-75}$, forced expiratory flow rate over the middle 50% of the FVC; FEF$_{50}$, forced expiratory flow after 50% of the FVC has been exhaled; FEV$_1$, forced expiratory volume in 1 second; FV, flow–volume; FVC, forced expiratory vital capacity; MVV, maximal voluntary ventilation; N, normal; PEF, peak expiratory flow; RV, residual volume; TLC, total lung capacity; ↓, decreased; ↑, increased.

3G • Nonspecific Pattern

About 18% to 20% of spirometry tests performed in our laboratory have a pattern suggestive of restriction, that is, reduced VC with normal FEV$_1$/FVC ratio. This is been called PRISm (preserved ratio impaired spirometry) by the COPDGene investigators.[7] In such cases, if lung volumes are measured, they confirm the impression of restriction in only about 50%. The other half has the curious combination of a reduced FVC with normal TLC and FEV$_1$/FVC ratio. Before 2009, there was no name for this pattern. That year we published a paper in which we named it the "nonspecific pattern" and described its characteristics (see Figure 3-8). Of patients with this pattern, 62% were men, over half had evidence of an obstructive disorder, despite the normal FEV$_1$/FVC ratio. Many had asthma. Obesity was common: 77% were overweight (BMI ≥ 25), 50% were obese (BMI ≥ 30), and 25% were very obese (BMI ≥ 35). Of the minority without obesity or asthma, we found patients with heart failure, muscle weakness, cancer, and chest wall abnormalities.[8] In a subsequent study, we found that the nonspecific pattern persists over 3 to 5 years of follow-up in 64% of individuals, while 16% evolve to restriction, 15% to obstruction, 3% to normal, and 2% to mixed pattern.[5] In unpublished data, we found that of patients with the NSP, 50% have increased airways resistance.

3H • Complex Restrictive Pattern

In typical restrictive disorders (e.g., interstitial disease), lung volumes are reduced proportionately. TLC and VC are reduced to similar degrees, and

RV may be either normal or reduced. It is not uncommon, however, to encounter a case of restriction in which the VC is reduced to a greater degree than the TLC, sometimes much greater. For example, TLC may be only mildly reduced at 72% predicted, while VC is severely reduced at 38% predicted. In such cases, the RV is increased, not decreased. What to make of such cases? Pulmonary function interpreters have argued whether to grade the severity of such restrictive cases based on TLC percent predicted or FVC percent predicted. Most use the former. In the above example, if using the TLC percent predicted, one would call it mild restriction, whereas if using the FVC percent predicted, one would call it severe restriction. Could this be mild-to-severe restriction? A few years back, I (PDS) considered this dilemma and with a brief review of such cases observed anecdotally that in the majority of such cases there was "something else" contributing to the reduction in FVC. That observation led to our study that describes the complex restrictive disorder. When FVC percent predicted is more than 10% smaller than TLC percent predicted, there is usually "something else," such as muscle weakness, chest wall limitation (including obesity), poor performance, or occult obstruction. RV/TLC is increased in both complex restriction and the nonspecific pattern (obstruction is not the only cause of high RV/TLC).[9] In many cases, measurements of maximal respiratory pressures are helpful. Also, such patients can often be further characterized by imaging or additional clinical assessments.

3I • Effect of Effort on FV Curve

This is an important topic that is often neglected. Figure 3-9 illustrates how variation in effort can affect the FV curve and hence the FEV_1 value.

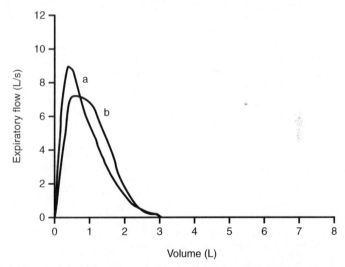

FIG. 3-9 Two consecutive maximal flow–volume curves. The effort was normal during curve a and the FEV_1 was 2.31 L. The effort during curve b was slightly less. This is reflected in the lower peak flow of 7.2 L/s. However, the FEV_1 of b was 2.70 L, which was 17% greater than curve a.

The patient produced two expiratory FV curves with equal exhaled volume, but the effort during curve b was less forceful. This is reflected in the lower peak expiratory flow (PEF). The surprising result is that the FEV_1 of curve b is 17% larger than that of a! Later, the patient produced two curves of equal effort with similar peak flows, and the FEV_1 values were now the same. This is the type of reproducibility of peak flows that provides the best reproducibility of the FEV_1.

PEF correlates well with the pleural pressure during the initial portion of the curve. In general, the higher the pleural pressure, the higher the PEF, and the more reproducible the FEV_1. The importance of being aware of this effort dependence of FEV_1 can come into play when evaluating the response to either a bronchoconstrictor or a bronchodilator agent (as discussed in Chapter 5). It is also important when comparing changes in the FEV_1 over time. There is a physiologic explanation for this apparent paradox of lesser effort resulting in greater flow. It has to do with differences in the initial degree of alveolar gas compression. To minimize this problem, aim for sharp peak flows in all FVC efforts. If you have several FVC efforts of nearly equal volumes, select the FEV_1 from the curve with the highest peak flow. This should give you the most reproducible FEV_1. Of additional importance is that this effort's effect is much greater in subjects with airway obstruction.[10]

PEARL Assume you had estimates of TLC by the plethysmographic method and a gas dilution method (nitrogen or helium). If the plethysmographic TLC exceeds that of the dilution method, you have an estimate of the volume of poorly ventilated lung, which is characteristic of airway obstruction. In Section 4B, page 40 (Pearl), another estimate of poorly ventilated volume is described when the D_{LCO} is measured.

PEARL What determines RV? As healthy adults and persons with obstruction exhale slowly and completely, airway resistance increases dramatically at low volumes as the airways narrow (see Fig. 7-4, page 69). When airway resistance approaches infinity, no further exhalation occurs and RV is reached. At this point, the small, peripheral airways are essentially closed. An increase in RV is sometimes the first sign of early airway disease. An exception to this description of how RV is determined can occur in children and young adults as well as persons with chest wall limitation. Their FV curve may show an abrupt cessation of flow with a contour similar to that seen in Figure 2-6E (page 14). An increase in airway resistance does not cause exhalation to cease. Rather, the respiratory muscles are not strong enough to compress the chest wall and abdomen any further. This increase in RV is not necessarily abnormal and usually disappears with growth and aging. For this reason, the term *air trapping* should be used with caution in persons with chest wall limitation.

REFERENCES

1. Gibson GJ. Lung volumes and elasticity. *Clin Chest Med* 22:623–635, 2001.
2. Miller RD, Offord KP. Roentgenologic determination of total lung capacity. *Mayo Clin Proc* 55:694–699, 1980.
3. Cotes JE, Chinn DJ, Reed JW. Body mass, fat percentage, and fat free mass as reference variables for lung function: effects on terms for age and sex. *Thorax* 56:839–844, 2001.
4. Olive JT Jr, Hyatt RE. Maximal expiratory flow and total respiratory resistance during induced bronchoconstriction in asthmatic subjects. *Am Rev Respir Dis* 106:366–376, 1972.
5. Iyer VN, Schroeder DR, Parker KO, Hyatt RE, Scanlon PD. The nonspecific pulmonary function test: longitudinal follow-up and outcomes. *Chest* 139:878–886, 2011.
6. Gardner ZS, Ruppel GL, Kaminsky DA. Grading the severity of obstruction in mixed obstructive-restrictive lung disease. *Chest* 140:598–603, 2011.
7. Wan ES, Castaldi PJ, Cho MH, Hokanson JE, Regan EA, Make BJ, Beaty TH, Han MK, Curtis JL, Curran-Everett D, Lynch DA, DeMeo DL, Crapo JD, Silverman EK. Epidemiology, genetics, and subtyping of preserved ratio impaired spirometry (PRISm) in COPDGene. *Respir Research* 15:89, 2014.
8. Hyatt RE, Cowl CT, Bjoraker JA, Scanlon PD. Conditions associated with an abnormal nonspecific pattern of pulmonary function tests. *Chest* 135:419–424, 2009.
9. Clay RD, Iyer VN, Reddy DR, Siontis B, Scanlon PD. The "Complex Restrictive" pulmonary function pattern: clinical and radiologic analysis of a common but previously undescribed restrictive pattern. *Chest* 152:1258–1265, 2017.
10. Krowka MJ, Enright PL, Rodarte JR, Hyatt RE. Effect of effort on measurement of forced expiratory volume in one second. *Am Rev Respir Dis* 136:829–833, 1987.

chapter 4

Diffusing Capacity of the Lungs

An important step in the transfer of oxygen from ambient air to the arterial blood is the process of diffusion, that is, the transfer of oxygen from the alveolar gas to the hemoglobin within the red cell. The pertinent anatomy is shown in Figure 4-1A. The path taken by oxygen molecules is shown in Figure 4-1B. They must traverse the alveolar wall, capillary wall, plasma, and red cell membrane and then combine with hemoglobin.

The diffusing capacity of the lungs (D_L) estimates the transfer of oxygen from alveolar gas to red cells. The amount of oxygen transferred is determined largely by three factors. One factor is the *area* (A) of the alveolar–capillary membrane, which consists of the alveolar and capillary walls. The greater the area, the greater the rate of transfer and the higher the D_L. Area is influenced by the number of blood-containing capillaries in the alveolar wall. The second factor is the *thickness* (T) of the membrane. The thicker the membrane, the lower the D_L. The third factor is the *driving pressure*, that is, the difference in oxygen tension between the alveolar gas and the venous blood (ΔPO_2). Alveolar oxygen tension is higher than that in the deoxygenated venous blood in the pulmonary artery. The greater this difference (ΔPO_2), the more oxygen transferred. These relations can be expressed as:

$$D_L \cong \frac{A \times \Delta PO_2}{T} \qquad \text{(Eq. 1)}$$

4A • The Diffusing Capacity for Carbon Monoxide

The diffusing capacity of oxygen (D_{LO_2}) can be measured directly, but this is technically extremely difficult. Measuring the diffusing capacity of carbon monoxide (D_{LCO}) is much easier and provides a valid reflection of the diffusion of oxygen. In essence, the difference between alveolar and venous carbon monoxide tension (ΔPCO) is substituted for the oxygen gradient in Eq. 1.

Several techniques for estimating D_{LCO} have been described. The most widely used is the single-breath (SB) method (SBD_{LCO}). The patient exhales to residual volume and then inhales a gas mixture containing a very low concentration of carbon monoxide (CO) plus an inert gas, such as helium. After a maximal inhalation, the patient holds his or her

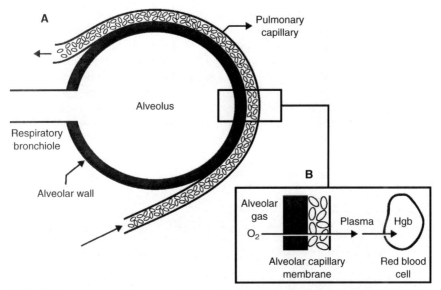

FIG. 4-1 A. Alveolar–capillary membrane through which oxygen must diffuse to enter the blood. In (B), alveolar wall is represented by the black rectangle. Hgb, hemoglobin.

breath for 10 seconds and then exhales completely. During the breath hold, CO is absorbed while helium equilibrates with alveolar gas. A sample of exhaled alveolar gas is collected and analyzed. By measuring the concentration of the exhaled CO and helium, the value of the DLCO can be computed. The helium is used to calculate the alveolar volume (VA), which is equal to the total lung capacity (TLC) minus anatomic dead space. The exhaled CO is used to calculate the amount of CO transferred to the blood.

DLCO is expressed in milliliters of CO absorbed per minute per mm Hg of driving pressure (the difference between partial pressure in alveolar gas and the blood).

The technical details of measurement of SBDLCO are complex. To improve accuracy and reproducibility of testing among laboratories, the American Thoracic Society and European Respiratory Society have established standards for performance of the test.[1]

4B • Normal Values of DLCO

An average normal value is 20 to 30 mL/min/mm Hg; that is, 20 to 30 mL CO is transferred per minute per mm Hg difference in the driving pressure of CO, namely, the difference between the partial pressure of CO in alveolar air and blood. The normal values depend on age (decrease with aging), sex (slightly lower in women), and size (taller people have larger lungs and therefore a higher DLCO).[2] The inclusion of helium provides an estimate of total V_A. D_{LCO}/V_A (perhaps better called carbon monoxide transfer coefficient [K_{CO}]) is often mistakenly thought of as "D_{LCO} adjusted for lung volume." In fact, K_{CO} is not constant with variations in lung volume at which it is measured. It increases in curvilinear fashion if measured at less than TLC. So in patients with restrictive lung diseases, it is not uncommon to have a normal K_{CO}. This should not be considered a "normal D_{LCO} adjusted for volume."[3]

With older pulmonary function equipment, some patients with small vital capacities were unable to exhale a sufficient quantity of the gas mixture to perform a valid test. Newer systems with rapid gas analyzers are able to perform valid measurements with most such test patients.

PEARL ● In the healthy patient, the V_A is nearly equal to TLC and can be used as an estimate of TLC. The V_A is also a good estimate of TLC in most restrictive conditions. In obstructive diseases, because of uneven distribution of ventilation, V_A underestimates TLC, just as the nitrogen washout and inert gas dilution techniques do (see Section 3C, page 26). The difference between TLC obtained with plethysmography and VA can be used as an estimate of the severity of nonuniform gas distribution, that is, the volume of poorly ventilated lung (see Chapter 3, first Pearl, page 26).

4C ● Causes of a Decreased D_{LCO}

Any process that decreases the surface area available for diffusion or thickens the alveolar–capillary membrane will decrease the D_{LCO} (Fig. 4-1B and Eq. 1). On the basis of these considerations, conditions that reduce the diffusing capacity can be determined (Table 4-1). The major ones are listed here.

Conditions That Decrease Surface Area

1. Emphysema: Although lung volume is increased, alveolar walls and capillaries are destroyed, and thus the total gas exchanging surface area is reduced. Reduction of the D_{LCO} in a patient with significant airway obstruction strongly suggests underlying emphysema.

2. Lung resection: If only a small portion of the lung is resected (such as a lobe in an otherwise healthy patient), capillary recruitment from the remaining normal lung can result in an equivalent gas exchanging surface area and capillary volume, and hence an unchanged D_{LCO}. If sufficient capillary surface area is lost, as with a pneumonectomy, the D_{LCO} is reduced.

3. Bronchial obstruction: A tumor obstructing a bronchus obviously reduces the area and lung volume. In an otherwise healthy lung, D_{LCO}/V_A may be increased.

TABLE 4-1   **Causes of a Decreased Diffusing Capacity**
Decreased *area* for diffusion
Emphysema
Lung/lobe resection
Bronchial obstruction, as by tumor
Multiple pulmonary emboli
Anemia
Increased *thickness* of alveolar–capillary membrane
Idiopathic pulmonary fibrosis
Congestive heart failure
Asbestosis
Sarcoidosis, involving parenchyma
Collagen vascular disease—scleroderma, systemic lupus erythematosus
Drug-induced alveolitis or fibrosis—bleomycin, nitrofurantoin, amiodarone, methotrexate
Hypersensitivity pneumonitis, including farmer's lung
Langerhans' cell histiocytosis (histiocytosis X or eosinophilic granuloma)
Alveolar proteinosis
Miscellaneous
High carbon monoxide back pressure from smoking
Pregnancy
Ventilation–perfusion mismatch

4. Multiple pulmonary emboli: By blocking perfusion to alveolar capillaries, emboli effectively reduce the area. Primary pulmonary hypertension causes a reduction in capillary area, but for unknown reasons does not consistently and reliably cause a reduction in D$_{LCO}$.

5. Anemia: By reducing pulmonary capillary hemoglobin, anemia also effectively reduces the area, as does any condition that lowers capillary blood volume. The usual adjustment for men with anemia is the following equation[1]:

$$D_{LCO}(cor) = D_{LCO}(unc) \times [10.22 + Hb] / [1.7 \times Hb] \quad (Eq.\ 2)$$

where cor represents corrected, unc represents uncorrected, and Hb represents hemoglobin. For women, the factor in the first set of brackets is 9.38 instead of 10.22.

Conditions That Effectively Increase Wall Thickness

As will be discussed in Chapter 6, much of the reduction in D$_{LCO}$ in the following conditions is also thought to be caused by mismatching of ventilation and perfusion.

1. Idiopathic pulmonary fibrosis, also called cryptogenic fibrosing alveolitis or usual interstitial pneumonia: It thickens the alveolar–capillary membrane and also decreases the lung volume.
2. Congestive heart failure: In this disorder, transudation of fluid into the interstitial space (tissue edema) or into the alveoli lengthens the pathway for diffusion.
3. Asbestosis: This is pulmonary fibrosis caused by exposure to asbestos.
4. Sarcoidosis: The granulomatous lesions may thicken the alveolar walls or cause distortion of microanatomy.
5. Collagen vascular disease: Conditions such as scleroderma and systemic lupus erythematosus probably alter or obliterate capillary walls, a situation that effectively increases the barrier to diffusion. This may be the first pulmonary function test result to become abnormal in these conditions.
6. Drug-induced alveolitis or fibrosis: Bleomycin, nitrofurantoin, amiodarone, and methotrexate are commonly associated with altered gas exchange.
7. Hypersensitivity pneumonitis: This condition includes farmer's lung.
8. Pulmonary Langerhans' cell histiocytosis, formerly called histiocytosis X or eosinophilic granuloma of the lung.
9. Alveolar proteinosis: Alveoli are filled with a phospholipid-rich material.

Miscellaneous Causes

1. The high CO tension in the blood of a heavy smoker can decrease the ΔPCO or driving pressure for CO. This lowers the D_{LCO} (Eq. 1).
2. Pregnancy has been reported to have various effects on D_{LCO} as a result of decreased hemoglobin, increased capillary blood volume, decreased lung volumes, and perhaps increased mismatching of ventilation and perfusion.
3. An isolated reduction in D_{LCO} (i.e., with normal results on spirometry and lung volumes) has been said to suggest pulmonary vascular disease, such as primary pulmonary hypertension, recurrent pulmonary emboli, or obliterative vasculopathy. However, a study of a cohort of such patients demonstrated that, in fact, this finding is more commonly seen in patients with emphysema or pulmonary fibrosis or both (so-called combined pulmonary fibrosis and emphysema).[4]

4D • Causes of Increased D$_{LCO}$

An increased D_{LCO} is not uncommon and usually not a matter of great concern. However, there are some interesting causes of an increased D_{LCO}. In a study of patients with a large D_{LCO} (>140% predicted), we found that the majority were obese or asthmatic or both, and so for most such patients, if there is evidence of asthma or obesity, a large DLCO probably does not warrant additional investigation.[5] Potential causes that can be considered include:

1. Asthma: Some patients with asthma, especially when symptom free, have an increased DLCO, possibly because the distribution of pulmonary blood flow is more uniform.
2. Obesity: The DLCO can be increased in obese persons, especially those who are massively obese. This increase is thought to result from an increased pulmonary blood volume.
3. Supine position: Rarely is the DLCO measured while the patient is supine, but this position produces a higher value because of increased perfusion and blood volume of the upper lobes.
4. Exercise or nonresting state: DLCO is increased because of increased pulmonary blood volumes.
5. Polycythemia: This is an increase in capillary red cell mass. This essentially amounts to an increase in area (A) in Eq. 1.
6. Intra-alveolar hemorrhage: In conditions such as Goodpasture syndrome, the hemoglobin in the alveoli combines with CO to produce an artificially high uptake of CO, which causes an increase in the calculated DLCO.
7. Left-to-right intracardiac shunt: This causes an increased pulmonary capillary volume.

Figures 4-2 through 4-4 present cases in which knowledge of the DLCO is very useful.

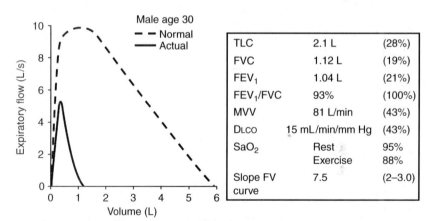

TLC	2.1 L	(28%)
FVC	1.12 L	(19%)
FEV$_1$	1.04 L	(21%)
FEV$_1$/FVC	93%	(100%)
MVV	81 L/min	(43%)
DLCO	15 mL/min/mm Hg	(43%)
SaO$_2$	Rest	95%
	Exercise	88%
Slope FV curve	7.5	(2–3.0)

FIG. 4-2 Case of severe restrictive disease. Total lung capacity (TLC) is markedly reduced, the ratio of forced expiratory volume in 1 second to forced vital capacity (FEV$_1$/FVC) is high, the carbon monoxide diffusing capacity of the lung (DLCO) is reduced, and the oxygen saturation (Sao$_2$) is decreased with exercise. The maximal voluntary ventilation (MVV) is not as severely reduced as the FEV$_1$; thus, the calculation of FEV$_1$ × 40 does not work in this situation. The steep slope of the flow–volume (FV) curve and the reduced DLCO suggest a pulmonary parenchymal cause of the severe restriction. The diagnosis in this case was idiopathic pulmonary fibrosis. Numbers in parentheses are percent of predicted, except for the slope of the FV curve, in which numbers indicate normal range.

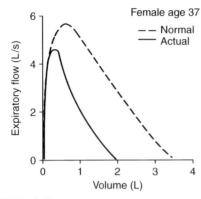

Female age 37		
TLC	3.35 L	(71%)
FVC	1.98 L	(57%)
FEV_1	1.70 L	(58%)
FEV_1/FVC	86.3%	(100%)
MVV	50 L/min	(45%)
DLCO	22 mL/min/mm Hg	(96%)
SaO_2	Rest	96%
	Exercise	94%
Slope FV curve	2.94	(2–3.0)

FIG. 4-3 As with Figure 4-2, this pattern is consistent with a restrictive process (reduced TLC, FVC, and FEV$_1$, and a normal FEV$_1$/FVC ratio). However, it differs from the case in Figure 4-2 in that the DLCO is normal, as is the slope of the FV curve. The MVV is also low. Further testing revealed a severe reduction in respiratory muscle strength (see Chapter 9), consistent with the diagnosis of amyotrophic lateral sclerosis. (Abbreviations and numbers in parentheses are defined in the legend to Fig. 4-2.)

4E • Other Considerations

The test for DLCO is very sensitive. With strict quality assurance, we have better reproducibility than published standards. The test-to-test variability in DLCO among our normal patients who test themselves regularly as part of our Biological QC Program is ±3.2 mL/min/mm Hg. We have found transient decreases of 3 to 5 mL/min/mm Hg with mild respiratory infections in healthy patients. It is a useful test for following the course of patients with idiopathic pulmonary fibrosis or sarcoidosis and for monitoring the toxicity of chemotherapy or for evaluating therapeutic interventions.

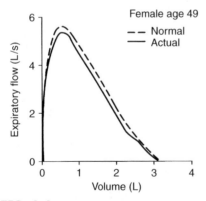

Female age 49		
TLC	4.81 L	(102%)
FVC	2.90 L	(92%)
FEV_1	2.37 L	(90%)
FEV_1/FVC	82%	(100%)
MVV	100 L/min	(100%)
DLCO	10 mL/min/mm Hg	(45%)
SaO_2	Rest	96%
	Exercise	90%
Slope FV curve	2.2	(2–3.5)

FIG. 4-4 In this case there is no apparent ventilatory limitation, the area under the FV curve being normal. All test values are normal except for the striking reduction in the DLCO and the desaturation with exercise. Primary pulmonary hypertension was diagnosed. (Abbreviations and numbers in parentheses are defined in the legend to Fig. 4-2.)

One might expect changes in the resting DLCO to be closely correlated with the arterial oxygen tension (PaO$_2$). However, this is not always so. For example, with lung resection larger than a lobe, DLCO is often reduced, but the PaO$_2$ is generally normal. However, a low resting DLCO often correlates with a decrease in PaO$_2$ during exercise.

PEARL • A reduced DLCO suggests a pulmonary vascular or parenchymal disorder. In a patient with a normal chest radiograph and no evidence of airway obstruction, this may indicate a need for further investigation, such as high-resolution computed tomography, to look for interstitial changes, or an echocardiography, to measure pulmonary artery pressure.

REFERENCES

1. Graham BL, Brusasco V, Burgos F, et al. 2017 ERS/ATS standards for single-breath carbon monoxide uptake in the lung. *Eur Respir J* 49(1), 2017. doi:10.1183/13993003.00016-2016.
2. Stanojevic S, Graham BL, Cooper BG, et al. Official ERS technical standards: Global Lung Function Initiative reference values for the carbon monoxide transfer factor for Caucasians. *Eur Respir J* 50(3), 2017. doi:10.1183/13993003.00010-2017.
3. Johnson DC. Importance of adjusting carbon monoxide diffusing capacity (DLCO) and carbon monoxide transfer coefficient (KCO) for alveolar volume. *Respir Med* 94:28–37, 2000.
4. Aduen JF, Zisman DA, Mobin SI, et al. Retrospective study of pulmonary function tests in patients presenting with isolated reduction in single-breath diffusion capacity: implications for the diagnosis of combined obstructive and restrictive lung disease. *Mayo Clin Proc* 82:48–54, 2007.
5. Saydain G, Beck KC, Decker PA, Cowl CT, Scanlon PD. Clinical significance of elevated diffusing capacity. *Chest* 125(2):446–452, 2004.

chapter 5

Bronchodilators and Bronchial Challenge Testing

Spirometry is often performed before and again after administration of an inhaled bronchodilator to assess responsiveness to such medications. A large degree of reversibility of obstruction is common in patients with asthma, whereas persistent irreversible obstruction is a defining feature of chronic obstructive pulmonary disease (COPD).[1,2] There is a large degree of overlap between conditions, so degrees of responsiveness are not reliably differentiated between conditions.

5A • Reasons for or Against Bronchodilator Testing

Administration of a β_2 agonist is rarely contraindicated. Ipratropium bromide can be administered in place of or in addition to a β_2 agonist. The major values of bronchodilator testing are as follows:

1. When testing for the first time, knowledge of both pre- and postbronchodilator values gives an idea of the range of impairment, at least at the time of testing. The degree of bronchodilator response has been correlated with clinical response to inhaled bronchodilator as well as susceptibility to acute exacerbations, rate of decline in lung function over time, and responsiveness to inhaled corticosteroid therapy.
2. COPD is defined by the presence of airflow obstruction that persists despite the administration of inhaled bronchodilator. According to COPD Guidelines, the degree of airflow limitation should be graded on the basis of postbronchodilator spirometry.
3. Bronchodilator response depends in part on the type and intensity of bronchodilator administered. The traditional dose of 2 puffs of

> **PEARL** ● Some pulmonologists believe that a positive response to a bronchodilator in COPD warrants a trial of inhaled corticosteroid therapy. However, bronchodilator response does not predict response to inhaled corticosteroid. Inhaled corticosteroid therapy is indicated for patients with moderate-to-severe COPD (forced expiratory volume in 1 second [FEV_1] <80% predicted) with frequent moderate (requiring steroids or antibiotics more than once a year) or any severe exacerbations (requiring hospitalization). This therapy reduces the frequency and severity of exacerbations and improves symptoms, lung function, and quality of life.[1,2]

albuterol typically results in a response that is minimal to modest in most patients with COPD. A larger dose (e.g., 4 puffs each of albuterol plus ipratropium bromide) results in a larger mean response and a larger proportion of individuals with a "positive" response.[3]

4. Bronchodilator responsiveness can vary from one test session to the next and is a poor predictor of clinical response to the use of bronchodilators. If no significant improvement occurs, a therapeutic trial (e.g., 2–4 weeks) of an inhaled bronchodilator in patients with obstructive disease may provide symptomatic and objective improvement.

5. An important finding may be the detection of unexpected responsiveness in a person with low-normal results on spirometry, which may lead to a diagnosis of unsuspected asthma.

5B • Administration of Bronchodilator

The agent can be administered either by a nebulizer unit or by the use of a metered-dose inhaler. The technique for the inhaler is described in Figure 5-1.

Ideally, the patient should not have used a bronchodilator before testing. Abstinence of 6 hours from inhaled short-acting β_2 agonists and anticholinergics and 12 to 24 hours from long-acting β_2 agonists (e.g., abediterol, arformoterol, formoterol, olodaterol, salmeterol, or vilanterol), anticholinergics (aclidinium, glycopyrrolate, revefenacin, tiotropium, or

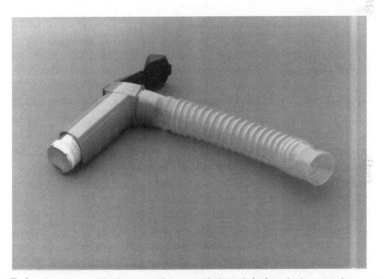

FIG. 5-1 Technique for the use of metered-dose inhaler. An inexpensive spacer of 5 to 6 inches is cut from disposable ventilator tubing. The patient is told to exhale toward residual volume, place the tubing in the mouth with lips around the tubing, and begin a slow, deep inspiration. The metered-dose inhaler is activated once at the start of inspiration, which continues to total lung capacity. The patient holds his or her breath for 6 to 10 seconds and then quietly exhales. After a few normal breaths, the procedure is repeated.

umeclidinium), and methylxanthines is recommended. The technician should always record whether the medications were taken and the time at which they were last taken. Use of corticosteroids need not be interrupted.

5C • Interpretation of Bronchodilator Response

The American Thoracic Society defines a significant bronchodilator response as one in which the FEV_1 or the forced expiratory vital capacity (FVC) or both increase by at least 12% and at least 200 mL.

> **PEARL** • An increase in FVC, which some call a *volume response*, may truly be caused by a reduction in air trapping but can also be caused by a prolonged expiratory effort in the absence of a real airway effect. To evaluate whether the increase in FVC is merely the result of a prolonged effort, compare the forced expiratory times and also overlay the control and postbronchodilator curves so that the starting volumes are the same, as in Figure 5-2B. If there is a slight increase in flow, then the increase in FVC is not caused by prolonged effort alone.

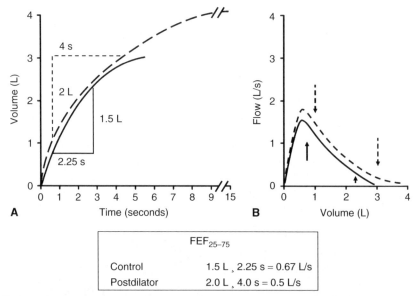

FEF$_{25-75}$	
Control	1.5 L ˏ 2.25 s = 0.67 L/s
Postdilator	2.0 L ˏ 4.0 s = 0.5 L/s

FIG. 5-2 **By definition, the FEF$_{25-75}$ (forced expiratory flow rate) is measured over the middle 50% of the vital capacity (A).** The spirograms and flow–volume curves show an increase in both flow and volume after use of a bronchodilator. Yet the control FEF$_{25-75}$ (0.67 L/s) is higher than the postdilator value (0.5 L/s). The reason for this apparent paradox can be appreciated from the flow–volume curves (B). The *solid arrows* indicate the volume range over which the control FEF$_{25-75}$ is calculated. The *dashed arrows* show the volume range over which the postdilator FEF$_{25-75}$ is calculated. The flows are lower at the end of the 25% to 75% volume range on the postdilator curve than those on the control curve. More time is spent at the low flows, which, in turn, causes the postdilator FEF$_{25-75}$ to be lower than the control value. Recommendation: Do not use the FEF$_{25-75}$ to evaluate bronchodilator response. Instead, use the FEV1 and FVC and *always* look at the curves.

The forced expiratory flow rate over the middle 50% of the FVC (FEF_{25-75}) is commonly said to be an indicator of small airways disease. However, it is not a useful indicator of airway obstruction and is *not* a reliable indicator of response to bronchodilator. A paradoxical decrease in FEF_{25-75} in response to bronchodilator is shown in Figure 5-2. Normal (negative) and abnormal (markedly positive) responses to inhaled bronchodilator are shown in Figure 5-3. Other examples are included in Chapter 15.

5D • Effect of Effort on Interpretation

In routine spirometry, changing effort can have a misleading effect on the FEV_1 and flow–volume curve. This has been discussed in Chapter 3, Section 3G. In Figure 5-4, the same patient has made two consecutive acceptable FVC efforts. During one effort (curve a), the patient made a maximal effort with a high peak flow and sustained maximal effort throughout the breath. However, in another effort (curve b), the patient exhaled with slightly less than the maximal force. The peak expiratory flow was slightly lower on curve b, but the flow on curve b exceeded that on curve a at lower volumes. The circles denote the FEV_1. In this

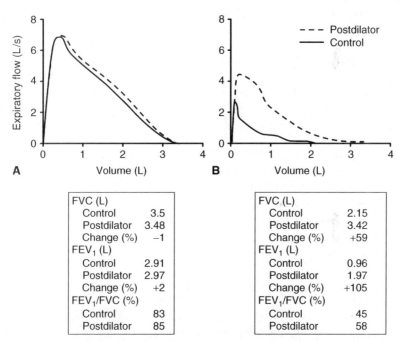

FVC (L)		
Control	3.5	
Postdilator	3.48	
Change (%)	−1	
FEV$_1$ (L)		
Control	2.91	
Postdilator	2.97	
Change (%)	+2	
FEV$_1$/FVC (%)		
Control	83	
Postdilator	85	

FVC (L)		
Control	2.15	
Postdilator	3.42	
Change (%)	+59	
FEV$_1$ (L)		
Control	0.96	
Postdilator	1.97	
Change (%)	+105	
FEV$_1$/FVC (%)		
Control	45	
Postdilator	58	

FIG. 5-3 Responses to inhaled bronchodilator. A. Normal response with −1% change in the forced expiratory vital capacity (FVC) and +2% change in the forced expiratory volume in 1 second (FEV_1). B. Markedly positive response with a 59% increase in the FVC and a 105% increase in the FEV_1. The FEV_1/FVC ratio is relatively insensitive to this change and therefore should not be used to evaluate bronchodilator response.

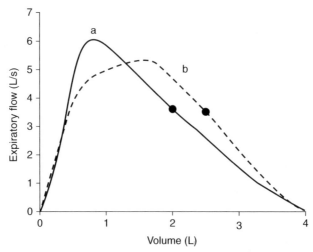

FIG. 5-4 Two consecutive flow–volume curves during which the patient exerted maximal effort (curve a) and then slightly submaximal effort (curve b). Note the slightly lower and delayed peak flow but higher flows over the lower volumes of curve b, which often results in an increased FEV_1. *Circles* indicate FEV_1 values.

situation, the slightly less forceful effort produced an FEV_1 of 2.5 L compared with 2.0 on curve a, a difference of 25%. This result could be interpreted as a significant bronchodilator effect had one been given. Clearly, the patient's lungs and airways have not changed, however.

There is a physiologic explanation for this apparent paradox, and the interested reader is referred to Krowka and associates.[4] It is important that one be alert to this potentially confusing occurrence, which can be substantial in patients with obstructive lung disease. The best way to minimize this problem is to require that all flow–volume curves have sharp peak flows, as in curve a in Figure 5-4, especially when two efforts are compared. Short of that, the peak flows should be very nearly identical ($<$10%–15% difference). The principle also applies to bronchial challenge testing (see below). This paradoxical behavior can easily be identified from flow–volume curves; it is almost impossible to recognize it from volume–time graphs.

5E • Indications for Bronchial Challenge Testing

The purpose of bronchial challenge testing is to detect patients with hyperreactive airways, a diagnostic feature of asthma, which is also found in patients with COPD. Although many patients with asthma present with typical features of wheezing, childhood atopy, chronic allergic features, and so on, some patients with asthma have atypical features, such as "cough variant asthma." For patients in whom clinical features are atypical, measurement of airway hyperresponsiveness may be helpful. Some indications for this procedure include the following:

1. To exclude or confirm a suspected diagnosis of asthma, for example, a history suggesting asthma with inconclusive results of spirometry with bronchodilator administration.
2. Chronic or episodic cough, chest tightness, or other atypical respiratory symptoms. Wheezing may be intermittently present but is not a required feature. Symptoms of asthma may be worse at night or after exercise or exposure to cold, dry, or polluted air.
3. Quantitative measures of airway responsiveness are sometimes used to assess degree of control and response to therapy.
4. Testing to assure absence of airway responsiveness in challenging environments such as military deployment, hazardous work environments, mountaineering, scuba diving, or others as deemed appropriate.
5. Consider cases of the *nonspecific pattern* (see Section 2F and reference 4 in Chapter 2) in which other cause (e.g., chest wall limitation, muscle weakness, and heart failure) is not apparent.

Contraindications include pregnancy, lactation, use of cholinesterase inhibitor medications (for myasthenia gravis), recent myocardial infarction or stroke (within 3 months), uncontrolled hypertension, aortic aneurism, recent eye surgery or increased intracranial pressure, respiratory compromise that could lead to respiratory failure with a too-vigorous response to challenge (e.g., $FEV_1 < 60\%$ predicted), and inability to perform acceptable and repeatable spirometry.

5F • Procedure for Bronchial Challenge Testing

The most commonly used agent for bronchoprovocation is inhaled methacholine, a direct cholinergic agonist drug that stimulates muscarinic receptors and causes contraction of smooth muscle in the airway. Histamine and other agents have been used in the past and for research studies, but methacholine is by far the most commonly used direct challenge agent. Other forms of bronchial challenge, such as exercise, cold air, osmotic or antigen challenge, rely on indirect mechanisms of bronchoconstriction. In either case, the degree to which the airways narrow depends on their reactivity, which is reflected in the magnitude of decrease in expiratory flow, usually quantified by measuring the FEV_1.

On exposure to an allergen, a person with asthma may experience an initial (within a few minutes) decrease in expiratory flow, which is called the *immediate* response. This is what is measured in bronchial challenge testing. It can be blocked by bronchodilators and cromolyn sodium. Some asthmatic individuals also experience a *late* or *delayed* response, which usually occurs 4 to 12 hours after exposure; it reflects the airway inflammatory response. This response can be blocked by corticosteroids or cromolyn sodium and is not elicited by methacholine. Inhaled allergens such as pollens may elicit either the early or the late responses or both. Although methacholine provokes only the early phase of the

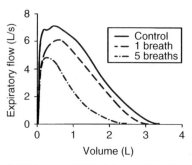

	Control	1 breath	5 breaths
FVC (L)	3.49	3.1	2.47
FEV$_1$ (L)	2.86	2.54	1.82
FEV$_1$ (% decrease)		11	36
FEV$_1$/FVC (%)	82	82	74

FIG. 5-5 Results of bronchial challenge testing in a 43-year-old woman who had a 3-year history of persistent cough, often at night. She denied wheezing but had mild dyspnea on exertion. One breath of methacholine produced a parallel shift in the flow–volume curve, no change in the ratio of forced expiratory volume in 1 second to forced expiratory vital capacity (FEV$_1$/FVC), a decrease of 11% in the FEV$_1$, and mild chest tightness. She was given four additional breaths of methacholine, and cough and chest tightness developed, but there was no audible wheezing. This is a positive test result with a 36% decrease in the FEV$_1$. Note that at five breaths, the flow–volume curve shows scooping and is no longer parallel with the control curve. The curve after one breath demonstrates that mild bronchoconstriction may produce only a mild decrease in FEV$_1$ and no change in the FEV$_1$/FVC ratio (see Section 3E, page 30 and Fig. 3-8A, page 32). Further constriction (curve after five breaths) leads to a flow–volume curve that is classic for obstruction, with scooping, a low FEV$_1$, and a decreased FEV$_1$/FVC ratio.

classic asthmatic hyperreactive airway response, it nevertheless is an excellent indicator of the presence of asthma. Thus, a positive result on methacholine challenge testing is predictive of asthma attacks that may be provoked by cold air, exercise, pollens, or viral infections. The lower the dose or concentration of methacholine that provokes a response, the greater the specificity of the test result. An example of a positive methacholine challenge study is illustrated in Figure 5-5.

Several protocols have been developed for bronchial challenge testing.[5] The most commonly used protocol is described in a recent technical standards paper.[6] After baseline spirometry is performed, a nebulized dose of diluent solution is administered, followed by a low dose of methacholine (e.g., 0.01 or 0.03 mg/mL) inhaled with a tidal breathing method or a deep breathing method or a shallow breathing method using a dosimeter. Spirometry is performed 1 and 3 minutes after each dose, and higher concentrations (either doubled or quadrupled) are administered every 5 minutes until a 20% decrease in FEV$_1$ is found or the highest dose is reached (16 mg/mL). From the available data, the concentration or dose at which FEV_1 decreases by 20% is calculated and reported. The technical standards paper recommends reporting the dose rather than the concentration at which the designated response occurs. However, calculation of dose requires specifications for nebulizer output and particle size distribution that are unavailable for most nebulizers. This makes calculation of PD20 the product of numerous "unknowns." There are a number of other controversies related to breathing method. The recommended tidal breathing method does not control for minute ventilation, which can vary by a factor of up to 4 among normal individuals, as anyone can attest who has monitored resting breathing by patients preparing for exercise testing.

Our laboratory performs most of our methacholine challenges using an abbreviated protocol similar to that described by Parker and associates[7] in 1965 and as used in the Lung Health Study.[8] The procedure is as follows:

1. Three milliliters of a 25 mg/mL solution of methacholine chloride in normal saline is placed in a standard nebulizer. It is not advisable to subject a patient to this abbreviated bronchial challenge if the baseline FEV_1 is less than 65% of predicted. If the FEV_1 is between 65% and 75% of predicted, the challenge is done starting with a lower concentration. If more reactive airways are suspected, a starting concentration of 5 or 1 mg/mL is used rather than 25 mg/mL. A lower concentration is also used in children, who are commonly more reactive.

2. Baseline spirometry is performed to obtain a reproducible FEV_1. The patient then inhales a breath of methacholine from the dosimeter, stopping inhalation short of a full breath to total lung capacity. The patient then holds his or her breath for 5 to 10 seconds and then breathes quietly.

3. Spirometry is repeated in 1 minute to obtain two reproducible measurements of FEV_1. Two or three efforts are performed and the best is reported. If the FEV_1 has decreased by 20%, the result is positive. If the FEV_1 has decreased by less than 15%, one breath of the next higher dose is administered. If the last dose was 25 mg/mL, four more breaths of 25 mg/mL methacholine are inhaled. If the decrease is between 15% and 19%, only two more breaths are inhaled.

4. Spirometry is repeated in 1 minute.

A response is *positive* if after the highest dose the FEV_1 is reduced by 20% or more of control value. In this case, a β_2 agonist is administered to reverse the effect of the methacholine. Although the final concentration is slightly higher than that used in the recommended protocol, the dose delivered is midway between the maximal doses of the recommended doubling protocol and the quadrupling protocol. It is possible to calculate a PD20 or PC20 from the protocol, but we report the result as simply positive (>20% response), borderline (15%–20% response) or negative (<15% response).

Technicians note whether the methacholine causes symptoms, such as chest tightness, substernal burning, cough, or wheezing. If the patient's symptoms are reproduced but the decrease in FEV_1 is borderline (15%–19%), we note that in the report.

Clinicians need to always be alert to the confounding effect of effort dependence on the FEV_1 (see Section 5D, page 49 and Fig. 5-4). For example, a control effort that is less than maximal may yield a value of FEV_1 that is falsely high compared with the value on a truly maximal effort after the inhalation of methacholine. A decrease in FEV_1 in this situation could be caused by varying effort and *not* hyperreactive airways. If the patient is incapable of performing acceptable baseline spirometry, we do not subject them to methacholine challenge, knowing the results would not be credible.

There are, of course, modifications to this approach that can be considered. For example, in a patient who becomes dyspneic or has chest tightness while cross-country skiing, cold air may be causing indirect bronchoconstriction. Baseline spirometry can be performed, after which the patient can exercise outside in the cold to reproduce the symptoms, and then a retest can be performed immediately or up to half an hour after the patient comes inside. The question of whether workplace exposure is causing symptoms can similarly be evaluated by testing before and immediately after a work shift. Laboratory challenges, such as exercise challenges, with or without cold or dry air exposure can attempt to mimic ambient conditions with varying degrees of success.

The following points need to be kept in mind:

1. Healthy patients may show a transient (for several months) increase in bronchial reactivity after viral respiratory infections, but they do not necessarily have asthma. This phenomenon is called the *postviral airway hyperresponsiveness syndrome.* It usually resolves spontaneously over about 6 weeks, but it also usually responds well to systemic or inhaled corticosteroid therapy, although commonly less so to inhaled bronchodilators.

2. In some persons with asthma, deep inspirations, such as those that occur with FVC maneuvers, can cause bronchoconstriction. This can lead to a progressive decrease in the FVC and FEV_1 on repeated efforts during routine testing, so-called *FVC induced bronchospasm.*

3. Likewise, a deep breath, either while inhaling methacholine or while performing spirometry, can have a bronchodilating effect, hiding the bronchoconstrictor effect of methacholine or other exposures. This can reduce the sensitivity of methacholine challenge. For this reason, the new challenge standard advises against coaching patients to inhale deeply during the administration of methacholine.

4. Patients with hyperreactive airways (i.e., a positive result on methacholine challenge test) may develop worsening

bronchospasm if given a nonselective β-adrenergic blocking agent. For example, this has been reported with the treatment of glaucoma using eye drops containing the nonselective β-adrenergic antagonist, timolol. On the other hand, selective β-blockers are often inappropriately withheld from patients with COPD or asthma, despite clear indications for coronary disease or hypertension, because of inappropriate fear of bronchospasm.

5. Many patients with COPD or chronic bronchitis have an increase in bronchial reactivity. There is considerable overlap between persons with asthma and those with COPD, leading to confusion in diagnosis and treatment.

6. Airway responsiveness may vary over time. It correlates with long-term control in asthma. It improves with long-term inhaled corticosteroid therapy. The degree of responsiveness correlates with the degree of airway narrowing because narrowed airways need to constrict only slightly to increase resistance and decrease the FEV_1 markedly.

5G • Exhaled Nitric Oxide in Laboratory Assessment of Asthma

Asthma is recognized as a disease characterized by airway obstruction, airway hyperresponsiveness to contractile stimuli, and airway inflammation. The challenges in the laboratory assessment of asthma are to identify evidence of inflammation or airway hyperresponsiveness in patients without baseline airway obstruction and to distinguish asthma as a cause of airway obstruction from other causes. Spirometry is helpful for grading the degree of airway obstruction both at baseline and after bronchodilator administration. Bronchoprovocation, most commonly with methacholine, is not always used, because there are safety issues for patients with moderate-to-severe obstruction and for certain other patients (e.g., pregnant women and patients with other medical conditions). Measures of airway inflammation are even less commonly used. Bronchial mucosal biopsy is invasive, and quantification of sputum eosinophils is challenging to perform accurately, although it has been standardized.[9]

For these reasons, an alternative assessment of airway inflammation could be helpful. Measurement of exhaled nitric oxide (NO) has been shown to correlate well with the presence of eosinophilic mucosal inflammation in patients with asthma.[10] NO was first described in exhaled breath in 1991. NO has been shown to be increased in most asthmatics and to be reduced by therapy with inhaled corticosteroids. It is also increased in viral respiratory tract infections, lupus erythematosus, hepatic cirrhosis, and lung transplant rejection. It is reduced or variable in COPD, cystic fibrosis, human immunodeficiency virus infection, and pulmonary hypertension.[11] It is decreased both acutely and chronically by cigarette smoking. Measurement of exhaled NO has been most widely applied for the diagnosis and management of asthma. The normal value for exhaled NO from the mouth is 3 to 7 parts per billion (ppb). The upper limit of normal, used to distinguish healthy persons from patients with asthma, has been variously reported between 15 and 50 ppb.

The method for measuring exhaled NO is somewhat complex and very dependent on a precise method for reproducible results. Care must be taken to maintain a stable airway pressure and expiratory flow rate and to avoid contamination with air from the nose and sinuses, which has a much higher concentration of NO. Methods have also been developed for measuring nasal exhaled NO as an indicator of sinusitis and allergic rhinitis. The American Thoracic Society and European Respiratory Society[12] published recommendations for standardized procedures for online and off-line measurements of exhaled lower respiratory tract NO and nasal NO in 2005.

There are several manufacturers of equipment for measuring NO. All equipment is based on chemiluminescence, a photochemical reaction of NO with ozone under high-vacuum conditions. A new Current Procedural Technology code, 95012, was approved by the American Medical Association in 2007 for billing for procedures. The role of measurement of exhaled NO in the diagnosis and management of asthma is evolving.

REFERENCES

1. GOLD. The Global Initiative for Chronic Obstructive Lung Disease [Homepage on the Internet]. Bethesda, MD: National Heart, Lung, and Blood Institute, National Institutes of Health, USA, and the World Health Organization [cited 2018 April 14]. Available from: http://goldcopd.org/wp-content/uploads/2017/11/GOLD-2018-v6.0-FINAL-revised-20-Nov_WMS.pdf.
2. Qaseem A, Wilt TJ, Weinberger SE, Hanania NA, Criner G, et. al. Diagnosis and Management of Stable Chronic Obstructive Pulmonary Disease: A Clinical Practice Guideline Update from the American College of Physicians, American College of Chest Physicians, American Thoracic Society, and European Respiratory Society. *Ann Intern Med* 155:179–191, 2011. http://www.thoracic.org/statements/resources/copd/179full.pdf.
3. Tashkin DP, Celli B, Senn S, et al. A 4-year trial of tiotropium in chronic obstructive pulmonary disease. *N Engl J Med* 359:1543–1554, 2008.
4. Krowka MJ, Enright PL, Rodarte JR, Hyatt RE. Effect of effort on measurement of forced expiratory volume in one second. *Am Rev Respir Dis* 136:829–833, 1987.
5. Crapo RO, Casaburi R, Coates AL, et al. Guidelines for methacholine and exercise challenge testing—1999. *Am J Respir Crit Care Med* 161:309–329, 2000.
6. Coates AL, Wanger J, Cockroft DW, et al. ERS technical standard on bronchial challenge testing: general considerations and performance of methacholine challenge tests. *Eur Respir J* 49(5), 2017. doi:10.1183/13993003.01526-201.
7. Parker CD, Bilbo RE, Reed CE. Methacholine aerosol as test for bronchial asthma. *Arch Intern Med* 115:452–458, 1965.
8. Tashkin DP, Altose MD, Bleecker ER, Connett JE, Kanner RE, et. al. The Lung Health Study: Airway Responsiveness to Inhaled Methacholine in Smokers with Mild to Moderate Airflow Limitation. *Am Rev Respir Dis* 145:301–310, 1992.
9. Pizzichini E, Pizzichini MM, Efthimiadis A, et. al. Indices of airway inflammation in induced sputum: reproducibility and validity of cell and fluid-phase measurements. Am J Respir Crit Care Med 154:308–317, 1996.
10. Payne DN, Adcock IM, Wilson NM, et al. Relationship between exhaled nitric oxide and mucosal eosinophilic inflammation in children with difficult asthma, after treatment with oral prednisolone. *Am J Respir Crit Care Med* 164:1376–1381, 2001.
11. Dweik RA, Boggs PB, Erzurum SC, et. al. An Official ATS Clinical Practice Guideline: Interpretation of Exhaled Nitric Oxide Levels (FENO) for Clinical Applications. *Am J Respir Crit Care Med* 184:602–615, 2011.
12. American Thoracic Society; European Respiratory Society. ATS/ERS recommendations for standardized procedures for the online and offline measurement of exhaled lower respiratory nitric oxide and nasal nitric oxide. *Am J Respir Crit Care Med* 171:912–930, 2005.

chapter 6

Arterial Blood Gases

Arterial blood gas analysis is performed to answer various clinical questions: Is gas exchange normal? If not, how bad is it? Is there hypoxemia (low oxygen saturation) at rest? Does the saturation decrease with exercise? Is there carbon dioxide retention in a patient with chronic obstructive pulmonary disease (COPD), severe asthma, or severe restrictive disease? What is the acid–base status?

Several important aspects need to be considered for obtaining and handling arterial blood specimens. The laboratory must always indicate on the report form whether the patient was breathing room air or an increased oxygen concentration. As stated in Section 3B (page 25), the arterial oxygen tension may be lower in the supine position than in an upright posture. Therefore, the posture of the patient should be noted. The patient should be neither hyperventilating nor holding his or her breath. The specimen should not contain any air bubbles, and it should be quickly iced and promptly analyzed. Similar precautions apply to the analysis of the pH of pleural fluid when empyema is a possibility.

6A • Arterial Oxygen Tension

There are four major steps in the transfer of oxygen from inhaled air to the tissues:

1. *Ventilation* of the alveoli must be adequate.
2. Within the lung, inhaled air must come in contact with venous blood; that is, there must be adequate *matching of ventilation* ($\dot{V}$) *to perfusion* ($\dot{Q}$).
3. There must be *diffusion* of oxygen through the alveolar wall into the hemoglobin in the red cells (see Chapter 4).
4. Oxygenated hemoglobin must then be transported by the cardiovascular system to the tissues.

The first two steps are discussed in this chapter. Transport, or so-called internal respiration, deals with the oxygen content of blood, the cardiac output, and the distribution of blood flow to the organs, topics that are outside the scope of this book.

The tension of oxygen in the arterial blood (Pa_{O_2}) reflects the adequacy of the transfer of oxygen from ambient air to blood. In healthy young adults, Pa_{O_2} values at sea level range from 85 to 100 mm Hg. The values decrease slightly with age, to about 80 mm Hg at age 70. *Hypoxemia* exists when the Pa_{O_2} is less than these values. The oxygen dissociation curve is useful in the consideration of hypoxemia. Figure 6-1

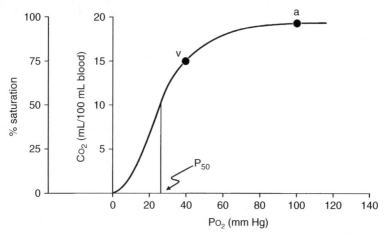

FIG. 6-1 **Oxyhemoglobin dissociation curve for hemoglobin that plots oxygen saturation against the partial pressure of oxygen (PO$_2$) and also the oxygen content (CO$_2$).** P$_{50}$ is the partial pressure of oxygen that results in a 50 saturation of hemoglobin. a, arterial blood; v, mixed venous blood. (From Taylor AE, Rehder K, Hyatt RE, et al., eds. *Clinical Respiratory Physiology.* Philadelphia, PA: W. B. Saunders, 1989. Used with permission.)

shows the average values for the oxygen tension of mixed venous blood (V ~ P$\bar{v}o_2$ = 40 mm Hg, saturation 75%) and arterial blood (a ~ Pao$_2$ = 100 mm Hg, saturation 96%). The curve is steep at and below the venous point, where small changes in oxygen tension produce dramatic change in the oxygen content of blood, and hence the saturation. Conversely, at oxygen tensions greater than 60 to 70 mm Hg, large changes in tension have a relatively small effect on saturation. Therefore, little additional oxygen can normally be added to the blood using high inspired oxygen tensions. Cyanosis is not easily appreciated until the saturation has decreased to less than 75%.

The four common causes of hypoxemia that occur with a *normal* inspired oxygen tension and barometric pressure are hypoventilation, ventilation–perfusion mismatch (V̇/Q̇), shunt, and impaired diffusion.

Hypoventilation

This term refers specifically to *alveolar* hypoventilation. There are two important, distinguishing features of alveolar hypoventilation. The first feature is that arterial carbon dioxide tension (Paco$_2$) is always increased. The following simple equation defines the relationship between Paco$_2$ and alveolar ventilation (V̇$_A$) and carbon dioxide production by the body (V̇$_{CO2}$) ("k" is a constant):

$$Paco_2 = k \times \frac{\dot{V}co_2}{\dot{V}_A} \quad (Eq.\ 1)$$

Assume $\dot{V}_{CO_2}$ stays constant. When $\dot{V}_A$ decreases, the $Paco_2$ must increase. Similarly, an increase in $\dot{V}_{CO_2}$ can increase $Paco_2$ unless alveolar ventilation increases proportionately.

A way to think of alveolar ventilation is as follows: When a patient inhales a tidal volume breath (designated V_T), a certain amount of that breath does not reach the gas-exchanging alveoli. A portion stays in the upper airway, trachea, and bronchi, and a portion may go to alveoli with no perfusion (especially in disease) so that gas exchange does not occur in either case. This fraction of the inhaled V_T is referred to as the dead space volume (VD). The VD is small in normal conditions but increased in diseases such as emphysema, chronic bronchitis, and acute respiratory distress syndrome (ARDS). If total ventilation ($\dot{V}_E$) is defined as the ventilation measured at the mouth, then

$$\dot{V}_A = \dot{V}_E - \dot{V}_E\left(\frac{V_D}{V_T}\right) \text{ (Eq. 2)}$$

Alveolar ventilation is the total ventilation minus the amount ventilating the dead space. Thus, $\dot{V}_A$ in Eq. 1 may be reduced by a decrease in V_E or by an increase in VD/V_T.

The second feature is that the hypoxemia due to alveolar hypoventilation can always be corrected by increasing the inspired oxygen concentration. An increase of approximately 1 mm Hg in inspired oxygen tension produces a 1-mm Hg increase in arterial oxygen tension. Inspired oxygen can be increased by several hundred millimeters of mercury, and hypoxemia is easily corrected. Some of the more common causes of hypoventilation are listed in Table 6-1; all reflect abnormalities in the function of the respiratory pump.

Hypoventilation can be identified as a cause of hypoxia with the use of the alveolar air equation:

$$Pao_2 = (Patm - Ph_2o)Fio_2 - \left(\frac{Paco_2}{RQ}\right) \text{ (Eq. 3)}$$

TABLE 6-1   Causes of Alveolar Hypoventilation

Central nervous system depression caused by drugs, anesthesia, and hypothyroidism
Disorders of the medullary respiratory center caused by trauma, hemorrhage, encephalitis, stroke, and tumor
Disorders of respiratory control such as sleep apnea and the obesity hypoventilation syndrome
Chest trauma with flail chest, kyphoscoliosis, and thoracoplasty
Neuromuscular disease affecting the efferent nerves (e.g., poliomyelitis, Guillain–Barré syndrome, and amyotrophic lateral sclerosis); the neuromuscular junction (e.g., myasthenia gravis); or the respiratory muscles (e.g., muscular dystrophy, acid maltase deficiency, and other myopathies)

where P_{AO_2} is the partial pressure of oxygen in the alveoli, P_{ATM} is the atmospheric pressure, P_{H_2O} is the partial pressure of water (47 mm Hg at body temperature), F_{IO_2} is the fraction of inspired oxygen, P_{ACO_2} is the partial pressure of carbon dioxide in the alveoli, and RQ is the respiratory quotient (usually 0.7–0.8 with a normal diet). P_{AO_2}–P_{aO_2} is usually called the A–a gradient or (A–a) DO_2. It is typically less than 10 in a young person and less than 20 in an older person. If it is normal, hypoxia is caused by hypoventilation or a low F_{IO_2}. If it is high, hypoxia may be caused by $\dot{V}/\dot{Q}$ mismatch, shunt, or diffusion impairment.

Ventilation–Perfusion Mismatch

Instead of the typical situation in which nearly equal volumes of air and venous blood go to all alveoli, a disparity (mismatch) may develop. Increased blood flow ($\dot{Q}$) may go to alveoli whose ventilation ($\dot{V}$) is reduced. Conversely, increased ventilation may go to areas with reduced blood flow. The result in either case is impaired gas exchange, often of a significant degree. In the ultimate hypothetical mismatch, all blood goes to one lung and all ventilation to the other, a situation incompatible with life. In the real-life situation, hypoxemia due to $\dot{V}/\dot{Q}$ mismatch can be improved and usually corrected by increased inspired oxygen concentrations.

$\dot{V}/\dot{Q}$ mismatch is the most common cause of hypoxemia encountered in clinical practice. It explains the hypoxemia in chronic bronchitis, emphysema, and asthma. It also explains much of the hypoxemia in interstitial lung disease and pulmonary edema.

Estimating the degree and type of mismatch is complex and beyond the scope of this book. Suffice it to say, an *increase* in the (A–a) DO_2 most often suggests the existence of lung regions with a low $\dot{V}/\dot{Q}$ ratio because perfusion exceeds ventilation. The so-called physiologic VD can also be estimated; an increase implies the existence of lung regions with a high $\dot{V}/\dot{Q}$ ratio due to a relative increase in ventilation. To pursue this interesting subject further, the reader should consult a standard text of respiratory physiology.

Right-to-Left Shunt

In this situation, a quantity of venous blood completely bypasses the alveoli. The shunt may be intracardiac, as in an atrial septal defect or tetralogy of Fallot, or it may occur within the lung, such as with arteriovenous fistulas in hereditary hemorrhagic telangiectasia (the Osler–Weber–Rendu syndrome). Blood flow through a region of total pneumonic consolidation or atelectasis also constitutes a right-to-left shunt. In shunt, the hypoxemia *cannot* be abolished by breathing 100% oxygen.

Impaired Diffusion

Diffusion is discussed in more detail in Chapter 4. As previously mentioned, $\dot{V}/\dot{Q}$ mismatch may contribute to the reduction in the diffusing capacity that is measured in a laboratory. Breathing a high-oxygen concentration can usually correct the hypoxemia caused by the diffusion impairment.

Mixed Causes

There are also mixed causes of hypoxemia. The patient with COPD and pneumonia has both $\dot{V}/\dot{Q}$ mismatch and right-to-left shunting. The patient with pulmonary fibrosis has both a diffusion defect and $\dot{V}/\dot{Q}$ mismatch.

6B • Arterial Carbon Dioxide Tension

The normal values for Pa_{CO_2} range from 35 to 45 mm Hg and, unlike Pa_{O_2}, are not affected by age. Figure 6-2 contrasts the dissociation curve of carbon dioxide with that of oxygen. The carbon dioxide curve does not have a plateau. Thus, the carbon dioxide content of blood is strongly dependent on Pa_{CO_2}, which in turn is inversely proportional to the level of alveolar ventilation (Eq. 1).

Hypercapnia (i.e., carbon dioxide retention with increased Pa_{CO_2}) can result from either of two mechanisms. The first mechanism, hypoventilation (Table 6-1), is more readily understood. Section 6A explains that Pa_{CO_2} is inversely proportional to alveolar ventilation (Eq. 1). When alveolar ventilation decreases, Pa_{CO_2} increases.

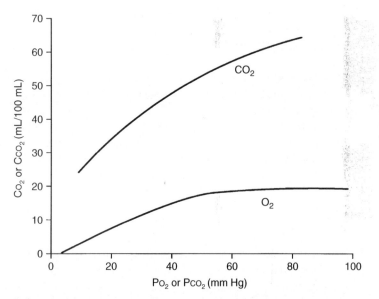

FIG. 6-2 Comparison of the shape of the oxyhemoglobin and carbon dioxide dissociation curves. The slope of the carbon dioxide dissociation curve is about three times steeper than that of the oxyhemoglobin dissociation curve. Cc_{O_2} is the carbon dioxide content of blood, C_{O_2} is the oxygen content of blood, and Pc_{O_2} and P_{O_2} are the partial pressures of carbon dioxide and oxygen in blood, respectively. (Modified from West JB, ed. *Respiratory Physiology: The Essentials*, 3rd ed. Baltimore, MD: Williams & Wilkins, 1985. Used with permission.)

The second mechanism, severe $\dot{V}/\dot{Q}$ mismatch, can also lead to carbon dioxide retention. When Pa_{O_2} decreases as a result of $\dot{V}/\dot{Q}$ mismatch, as discussed previously, Pa_{CO_2} increases. This commonly occurs in COPD. However, in some patients, ventilation increases to maintain a normal Pa_{CO_2}. Pa_{O_2} also improves some. These are the "pink puffers." In other patients with COPD, the Pa_{CO_2} increases and the Pa_{O_2} decreases as a result of $\dot{V}/\dot{Q}$ mismatch. These are the classic "blue bloaters," the cyanotic hypoventilators. Of course, many patients with COPD have a course between these two extremes.

6C • Arterial pH

pH is the negative log of the hydrogen ion concentration. This means that in acidosis (low pH), there is an increase in H^+ ions. The converse holds for alkalosis, with its decrease in H^+ ions and increased pH.

The acid–base status of blood is classically analyzed in terms of the Henderson–Hasselbalch equation for the bicarbonate buffer system, which highlights the importance of the arterial partial pressure of carbon dioxide (P_{CO_2}).

$$pH = pK + \log \frac{[HCO_3^-]}{0.03\ P_{CO_2}} \text{ (Eq. 4)}$$

The pK is a constant related to the dissociation of carbonic acid. Note that with constant bicarbonate, increases in the P_{CO_2} lower the pH. Conversely, lowering the P_{CO_2} by increasing ventilation produces alkalosis (increased pH).

Respiratory alterations in acid–base status are related to elimination of carbon dioxide. Metabolic abnormalities, however, entail either a gain or a loss of fixed acid or bicarbonate in the extracellular fluid. Metabolic alterations in acid–base balance can be rapidly compensated for by alternating the amount of carbon dioxide eliminated by ventilation. This is followed by the slower elimination by the kidneys of excess acid or base.

The Davenport pH–[HCO_3^-] diagram shown in Figure 6-3 is a useful way of looking at the body's response to acid–base alterations. It is a graphic representation of the Henderson–Hasselbalch equation. Shown are three different buffer lines (slanting down and to the right) defining the [HCO_3^-] and pH responses, resulting from adding metabolic acid or base to plasma. Also shown are three isopleths (slanting up and to the right) relating pH to [HCO_3^-] for three levels of P_{CO_2}. Point A indicates the normal situation: pH = 7.4, [HCO_3^-] = 24 mEq/L, and P_{CO_2} = 40 mm Hg.

Compensatory Mechanisms

1. Respiratory acidosis: Point B in Figure 6-3 shows the result of acute hypoventilation; P_{CO_2} increases and pH decreases. The kidney seeks to compensate for the acidosis when hypoventilation becomes

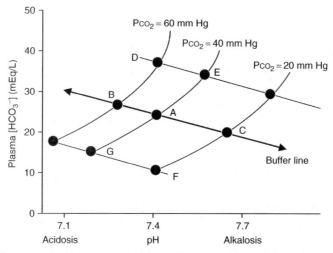

FIG. 6-3 Davenport diagram showing [HCO$_3^-$] as a function of pH and partial pressure of carbon dioxide (Pco$_2$). (From Taylor AE, Rehder K, Hyatt RE, et al., eds. *Clinical Respiratory Physiology*. Philadelphia, PA: W. B. Saunders, 1989. Used with permission.)

chronic, as in COPD, by conserving [HCO$_3^-$]. The result is that point B moves toward point D and pH returns toward normal.

2. Respiratory alkalosis: Point C shows what occurs with acute hyperventilation; Pco$_2$ decreases and pH increases. As hyperventilation persists, for example, during acclimatization to altitude, the kidneys excrete [HCO$_3^-$], and as predicted from Eq. 2, the pH is normalized from C toward F.

3. Metabolic acidosis: Point G represents acidosis due to the accumulation of fixed acids with a lowering of plasma [HCO$_3^-$]. The respiratory system attempts to compensate for this by increasing ventilation, thus lowering Pco$_2$ and moving from G toward F. The classic example is the hyperpnea of diabetic ketoacidosis.

4. Metabolic alkalosis: Loss of fixed acids, as with repeated vomiting, causes a shift from A to E. The respiratory response is a decrease in ventilation, resulting in an increase in Pco$_2$ and movement from E toward D.

6D • An Alternative Approach to Acid–Base Analysis

An alternative approach to the Davenport diagram is preferred by some and may be easier to use in the community hospital setting. Not all laboratories that perform arterial blood gas analysis have a co-oximeter to determine the bicarbonate level. The bicarbonate level can be calculated with the Henderson equation, in which [H$^+$] is the hydrogen ion concentration:

$$[H^+] = 24 \times \frac{Pco_2}{[HCO_3^-]} \quad \text{(Eq. 5)}$$

This can be rearranged to calculate the bicarbonate concentration:

$$[HCO_3^-] = 24 \times \frac{Pco_2}{[H^+]} \quad (Eq.\ 6)$$

The $[H^+]$ (in mEq) can be calculated from the pH. Typical values are listed in Table 6-2. Intermediate values can be calculated by interpolation. Once the bicarbonate, the pH, and the Pco_2 values are found, the acid–base status can be determined, and respiratory and metabolic causes of acidosis and alkalosis can be distinguished, as discussed in Section 6C and Figure 6-3. A complete discussion of acid–base disturbances is beyond the scope of this book.

6E • Additional Considerations

Many blood gas laboratories use a co-oximeter to measure total hemoglobin (Hb), Hb saturation, carboxyhemoglobin (COHb), and methemoglobin (MetHb) and to calculate bicarbonate and arterial oxygen-carrying capacity (Cao_2). In the emergency department, measurement of COHb and MetHb is valuable for detecting carbon monoxide poisoning and toxicity from various medications that cause methemoglobinemia. In the intensive care unit, arterial blood gas values are checked frequently, and co-oximeter results often provide the first sign of blood loss in patients who have a high risk of gastrointestinal hemorrhage.

Mandated procedures and inspections under the Clinical Laboratories Improvement Act have improved quality control in arterial blood gas laboratories. Physicians should be aware of issues related to sample contamination and calibration of medical instrumentation. A useful rule is that the sum of the Pco_2 and partial pressure of oxygen (Po_2) should not exceed roughly 150 mm Hg with the patient breathing room air. If the sum is greater than this, either the patient is breathing supplemental oxygen or the instrument's calibration needs to be checked.

TABLE 6-2 Relation of pH to Hydrogen Ion Concentration	
pH	[H⁺]
7.50	32
7.40	40
7.30	50
7.22	60
7.15	71
7.10	79
7.05	89
7.00	100

6F • Some Possible Problems

CASE 1

The following blood gas results are from a 40-year-old patient who was sitting when the arterial blood was drawn:

$$Pao_2 = 110 \text{ mm Hg}$$

$$Paco_2 = 30 \text{ mm Hg}$$

$$pH = 7.50$$

Question

How should these results be interpreted, and what is the underlying problem?

Answer

The data indicate uncompensated acute respiratory alkalosis. The patient was frightened by the needle and hyperventilated as the blood was drawn.

CASE 2

The patient is a small, 70-year-old woman with lobar pneumonia. The Pao_2 value on admission was 50 mm Hg and saturation was 80%; she was given 40% inspired oxygen. Two hours later, the patient looked somewhat better, but the Pao_2 value was not improved. However, when the saturation was measured by pulse oximetry, it had increased to 92%.

Question

What might be the cause of the disparity between the blood gas and oximetry data? If the blood gas study was correct, intubation was indicated.

Answer

The technician was asked to draw another blood sample while saturation was monitored by pulse oximetry. As this was done, it was obvious that the patient held her breath during the needle-stick and blood sampling and saturation decreased. Because of her small lung volumes, further reduced by pneumonia, her alveolar oxygen tension decreased drastically, leading to the low Pao_2. In a sample drawn when she did not hold her breath, the Pao_2 was 80 mm Hg and the saturation was 92%.

CASE 3

A 55-year-old man is being evaluated for weakness and chronic cough. He has had progressive difficulty swallowing for 6 months. His chest radiograph shows small lung volumes and bibasilar atelectasis with a superior segment infiltrate in the left lower lobe. P_{O_2} is 45 mm Hg breathing room air, and P_{CO_2} is 62 mm Hg.

Question

What is the cause of his hypoxia?

Answer

Hypoventilation due to respiratory muscle weakness (see Chapter 9). The A–a gradient is nearly normal. Despite the radiographic abnormalities, his $\dot{V}/\dot{Q}$ matching is still good. He is hypoxic because of his hypercapnia.

chapter 7

Other Tests of Lung Mechanics: Resistance and Compliance

The tests described here are usually performed in fully equipped clinical laboratories or research laboratories. In the outpatient setting, they add relatively little to the basic evaluations discussed in previous chapters (spirometry, lung volumes, diffusing capacity, and arterial blood gases). However, these tests might be encountered in either specialty graduate training or in laboratory reports and, therefore, are considered briefly. Perhaps more importantly, understanding these concepts is important in the management of patients requiring mechanical ventilation.

7A • Resistance

Resistance is the pressure required to produce a flow of 1 L/s into or out of the lung. The units are centimeters of water per liter per second (cm $H_2O/L/s$). This general concept is illustrated in Figure 7-1, in which the

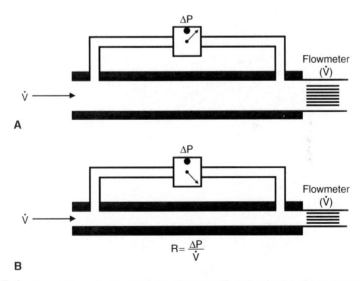

FIG. 7-1 Measurement of resistance (R) through a large tube (A) and small tube (B). Flow ($\dot{V}$) is measured by the flowmeter, and driving pressure (ΔP) is measured by a differential pressure transducer. To drive the same flow requires a greater pressure in tube (B) and hence the R of tube (B) is higher than that of tube (A).

pertinent driving pressure (ΔP) is the pressure difference between the ends of the tubes. The pressure required to produce a flow of 1 L/s in a large tube is less than that required in a small tube. Hence, the resistance (R) of the small tube is much higher than that of the large tube.

In the lung, measurement of the resistance of the entire system is of interest. Figure 7-2 illustrates how this can be obtained. Flow at the mouth can be measured with a flowmeter. The pressure driving the flow can be measured in either of two ways. Pleural pressure (Ppl) can be measured using a small balloon–tipped catheter unit placed in the lower third of the esophagus and attached to a pressure transducer. Pressure changes in the esophagus have been shown to reflect those in the pleural cavity. The difference between Ppl and Pao (the pressure at the mouth) is the driving pressure. Dividing the driving pressure by flow ($\dot{V}$) yields pulmonary resistance (Rpulm). Rpulm includes airway resistance (Raw) plus a small component due to the resistance of the lung tissue.

The other, more commonly used, resistance measurement is obtained by measuring alveolar pressure (Palv) in relation to Pao. Palv can be measured in a body plethysmograph and does not require swallowing an esophageal balloon. In this method, the driving pressure is Palv − Pao. This result is divided by flow to determine Raw. Raw is slightly lower than Rpulm because of the absence of tissue resistance. Both Rpulm and Raw can be measured during either inspiration or expiration, or as an average of both. Figure 7-3 describes how Raw is measured.

Average resistance in normal adults is 1 to 3 cm H_2O/L/s. It is higher in the small lungs of children because their airways are smaller. Occasionally, the term *conductance* is used. Conductance is a term borrowed from the electrical engineering field and is the reciprocal of resistance; its

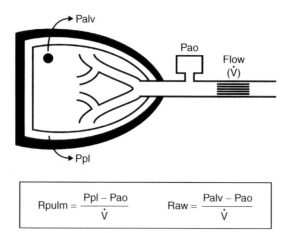

$$Rpulm = \frac{Ppl - Pao}{\dot{V}} \qquad Raw = \frac{Palv - Pao}{\dot{V}}$$

FIG. 7-2 Model illustrating how pulmonary resistance (Rpulm) and airway resistance (Raw) are measured. An esophageal balloon is required to measure pleural pressure (Ppl), whereas Palv can be inferred from noninvasive measures in body plethysmography. Palv, alveolar pressure; Pao, pressure at the mouth; $\dot{V}$, flow.

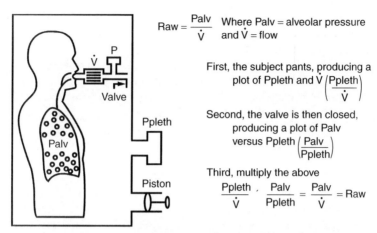

FIG. 7-3 The equipment used to measure lung volume by the body plethysmo-graph (see Fig. 3-6, page 29) has been modified by inserting a flowmeter between the patient's mouth and the pressure gauge and valve. The flowmeter measures airflow ($\dot{V}$). The patient is instructed to pant shallowly through the system with the valve open. This provides a measure of plethysmographic pressure as a function of flow, that is, Ppleth/$\dot{V}$ (see bottom equation). With the patient still panting, the valve is closed. This provides a measure of alveolar pressure as a function of plethysmographic pressure, that is, Palv/Ppleth (also in bottom equation). As shown, airway resistance (Raw) is obtained by multiplying these two ratios.

units are liters per second per centimeter of water, L/s/cm H_2O. Thus, a high resistance means a low conductance—flow is not "conducted" well.

Resistance varies inversely with lung volume (Fig. 7-4). At high lung volumes, the airways are wider and the resistance is lower. Conversely, at

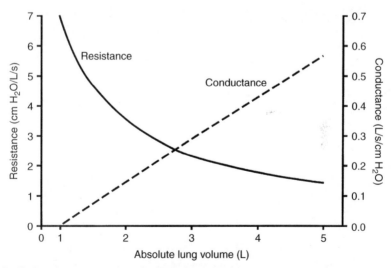

FIG. 7-4 Resistance is a hyperbolic function of lung volume. When its reciprocal, conductance, is plotted, a straight line results. Note that the conductance line intersects the volume axis at 1 L, which is the residual volume in this example. At that point, conductance reaches zero, and its inverse, resistance, approaches infinity.

low lung volumes, resistance increases until the point of airway closure at residual volume. To standardize for this effect, resistance is typically measured during breathing at functional residual capacity.

Resistance is increased when the airways are narrowed. Narrowing may be caused by smooth muscle contraction, bronchial wall thickening from inflammation, or mucus production, all features of asthma and chronic bronchitis, floppy airways (as in emphysema), or mechanical obstruction (as in lung cancer or an aspirated foreign body).

There is a strong negative correlation between resistance and maximal expiratory flow (V̇max). A high resistance is associated with decreased flows, as indicated by decreases in the forced expiratory volume in 1 second (FEV_1) and other flows such as the forced expiratory flow at 25% to 75% of the pulmonary volume (FEF_{25-75}). There are, however, a few exceptions to this relationship. One is illustrated in Figure 7-5. This type of V̇max–volume curve is occasionally seen in the elderly. Resistance in this case is normal, but flows at low lung volumes are reduced. This is why age-adjusted values for spirometry reference values, particularly the FEV_1/FVC (forced vital capacity) ratio, are important (rather than using an arbitrary threshold of 0.7 for the lower limit for the FEV_1/FVC ratio).

PEARL ● A patient with a variably obstructing lesion in the extrathoracic (upper) trachea (see Fig. 2-7D, page 16) may have a considerable increase in airway resistance but normal V̇max. The increased resistance reflects the markedly decreased inspiratory flows caused by the high inspiratory resistance. Separate calculations of inspiratory and expiratory resistance make this obvious.

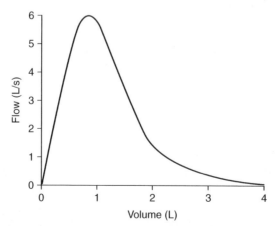

FIG. 7-5 **Flow–volume curve showing normal flow at high lung volumes but abnormally low flows over the lower 50% of vital capacity.** In this case, resistance is often normal, but the forced expiratory flows at low lung volumes are reduced.

7B • Pulmonary Compliance

Compliance is a measure of the lungs' elasticity. Compliance of the lungs (C_L) is defined as the change in lung volume resulting from a change of 1 cm H_2O in the elastic pressure of the lungs. Figure 7-6 is similar to Figure 7-2, but a spirometer is added to measure volume (V). When the lung is not moving (i.e., airflow is zero), the Ppl is negative (subatmospheric). The lungs are elastic and tend to collapse. This is resisted by the chest wall, so the Ppl, when volume is not changing, reflects the static elastic pressure or recoil of the lung at that volume. If lung volume is increased by a known amount (ΔV) and volume is again held constant, the new Ppl is more negative (the recoil of the lung is greater). This ΔV divided by the difference in the two *static* Ppl values (ΔPpl) defines the lung compliance, $C_L = \Delta V/\Delta Ppl$ (L/cm H_2O) at that volume. In addition, it is common practice to measure the elastic recoil pressure with the patient holding his or her breath at total lung capacity (TLC); this is termed the *PTLC* (recoil pressure at TLC). The measurement of C_L requires the introduction of an esophageal balloon to measure Ppl. Interest in this physiology has increased because some mechanical ventilators now incorporate the measurement of esophageal pressure into their advanced diagnostics.

Compliance measured when there is no airflow, as in the foregoing discussion, is termed *static compliance* ($C_{L_{stat}}$). Compliance is often measured during quiet breathing and with an esophageal balloon–catheter system. During a breath, there are two times when airflow is zero: at the end of inspiration and at the end of expiration. The difference in Ppl at these two times also defines a change in elastic recoil pressure. This ΔPpl divided into the ΔV is called the dynamic compliance of the lung ($C_{L_{dyn}}$).

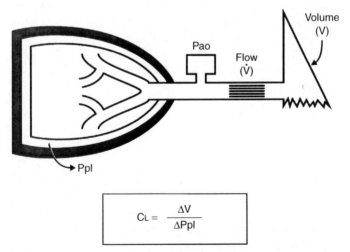

$$C_L = \frac{\Delta V}{\Delta Ppl}$$

FIG. 7-6 Model demonstrating the measurement of compliance. An esophageal balloon is required. CL, compliance of the lungs; Pao, pressure at the mouth; Ppl, pleural pressure.

In normal adult patients, CL_{stat} and CL_{dyn} are nearly the same and range from 0.150 to 0.250 L/cm H_2O. CL varies directly with lung size, with compliance being lower in patients with small lungs.

Compliance is reduced in patients with pulmonary fibrosis, often to values as low as 0.050 L/cm H_2O, reflecting the fact that these lungs are very stiff. Large changes in pressure produce only small changes in volume. Again, static and dynamic compliance are similar.

The situation in chronic obstructive pulmonary disease (COPD), especially emphysema, is different. Static compliance is increased, often to values more than 0.500 L/cm H_2O. This high compliance reflects the floppy, inelastic lungs. However, CL_{dyn} is much lower, often in the normal range. The explanation for this apparent paradox relates to the nonuniform ventilation of the lungs in COPD, as will be discussed in Chapter 8. In essence, during breathing in COPD, air preferentially flows into and out of the more normal regions of the lung. Because the elasticity of these regions is not as severely impaired, CL_{dyn} is closer to normal values. This difference between CL_{stat} and CL_{dyn} is referred to as frequency dependence of compliance. It is important to remember that a low CL_{dyn} in COPD does not mean that the lung is stiff or fibrotic.

7C • Respiratory System Compliance

The compliance of the entire respiratory system (Crs) can also be measured. It requires that the respiratory muscles be relaxed. This measurement is most often made when a patient is on a ventilator. The patient's lungs are inflated, the airway is occluded, and the occluded airway pressure is measured. The lungs are allowed to deflate a measured amount, and a second occlusion pressure is obtained. Crs is the change in volume divided by the difference in the two pressures. Because the lungs and chest wall are in series, Crs includes both lung (CL_{stat}) and chest wall (Ccw) compliance. Because the reciprocals of the compliances are added, the equation describing this relationship is as follows:

$$\frac{1}{Crs} = \frac{1}{CL_{stat}} + \frac{1}{Ccw} \quad (Eq. 1)$$

Thus, a decrease in Crs may be caused by a decrease in either CL_{stat} or Ccw compliance (or both), a fact that is sometimes overlooked. This is critically important in the intensive care unit, where an increase in the pressure required to ventilate a patient may result from an increase in lung stiffness or from an inadequately sedated patient. It is also worth noting that sometimes calculations are easier to comprehend using elastance (E), which is 1/C. For example, Ers = EL_{stat} + Ecw.

7D • Pathophysiology of Lung Mechanics

The basics of lung mechanics have been presented. This section details the mechanical handicaps associated with obstructive and restrictive lung diseases.

Lung Static Elastic Recoil Pressure

We noted previously that the Ppl measured when the lung is not moving is the static elastic recoil pressure of the lung, which we now define as Pst. This pressure is measured with a small balloon–tipped catheter placed in the lower esophagus.

In Figure 7-7, Pst is plotted during deflation of the lung from TLC to residual volume. Three cases are shown: a healthy patient (N); a patient with emphysema, an obstructive disorder (E); and a patient with pulmonary fibrosis, a restrictive disease (F). The curves are plotted as a function of absolute lung volume. Note the loss of lung recoil and hyperinflation in emphysema (E). This contrasts with the reduced lung volume and increased lung recoil in pulmonary fibrosis (F).

The E curve emphasizes two problems faced by the patient with emphysema and by most patients with COPD. First, the loss of recoil pressure means that the lung parenchyma cannot distend the airways as much as in the normal case (see the tethering springs in Fig. 2-2, page 6). Second, as shown in Figure 9-2 (page 83), the ability of the inspiratory muscles to generate force is reduced because of hyperinflation.

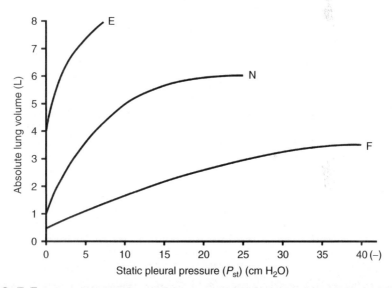

FIG. 7-7 Lung static elastic recoil pressure (Pst) is plotted against absolute lung volume for three typical patients: a patient with emphysema (E), a healthy patient (N), and a patient with pulmonary fibrosis or acute respiratory distress syndrome (ARDS) (F). Although pleural pressure is negative, it is usually plotted to the right, as shown.

In the F curve, representing the patient with pulmonary fibrosis (or ARDS [acute respiratory distress syndrome]), the ability of the expiratory muscles to develop force is reduced (see Fig. 9-2, page 83) because of the reduced lung volume. In addition, the increased recoil of the fibrotic or inflamed lung requires the respiratory muscles to exert greater than normal force to expand the lung.

PEARL ● You might think that the Pst derives from the elastic and collagen fibers in the healthy lung. However, the major contribution of elastic recoil comes from surface tension forces acting at the air–fluid interface in the alveoli. This is demonstrated in Figure 7-8, in which plotted static inflation and deflation airway pressures in a lung contain air (the normal situation), and the same lung is inflated and deflated with saline after the air has been removed. With saline filling the lung, the air–fluid interface in the alveoli is abolished, and the surface tension is eliminated with it. Note how little recoil pressure remains in the saline-filled lung, which reflects the small tissue contribution. The large difference between inflation and deflation curves represents hysteresis—a common property of biologic tissues.

Work of Breathing

Figure 7-9 illustrates the effects of the alterations in Pst and in airflow resistance on the work of breathing required of the respiratory muscles. The static curves of Figure 7-7 have been replotted; the Ppl during inspiration

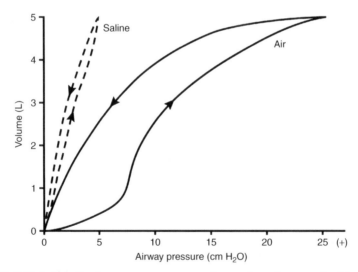

FIG. 7-8 Plot of static airway pressure versus lung volume in an excised lung first inflated and deflated with air. The *arrows* indicate the inflation and deflation paths. The lung is then degassed (all air is removed) and inflated and deflated with saline. The marked shift to the left of the saline curve reflects the loss of recoil when surface tension at the alveolar air–fluid interface is eliminated. The difference between the inflation and deflation curves is called hysteresis.

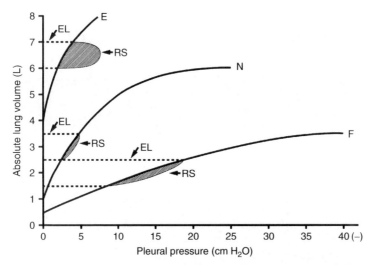

FIG. 7-9 **The negative pleural pressure generated during an inspiratory breath is plotted for a healthy patient (N), a patient with emphysema (E), and a patient with fibrosis (F).** The inspiratory loops are plotted on the static recoil curves of Figure 7-7. The hatched areas reflect the work of breathing required to overcome the resistance to airflow (RS). The areas between the static curve and the zero-pressure line reflect the work required to keep the lung inflated, the elastic work (EL). See text for further discussion.

has been added to each curve. Work is a product of pressure and volume (the area of the V vs. P loop). In each case, the hatched area between the inspiratory loop (identified by the *arrows*) and the static curve represents the resistive work (RS) of that breath. It is increased in the E curve. The area between the static curve and the zero-pressure axis reflects the work required to keep the lung inflated, that is, the elastic work (EL). Compared with the normal curve, the patient with emphysema has increased work because of increased airflow resistance, whereas the patient with fibrosis or ARDS has increased EL because of the stiffness of the lung. Although the total inspiratory work loop is less in emphysema than in fibrosis, more work is required during expiration. In addition, the hyperinflation in emphysema puts the system at a distinct mechanical disadvantage.

Static Lung Recoil Pressure and Maximal Expiratory Flow

In Section 2B (page 5) and Figure 2-2 (page 6), we noted that lung elasticity, specifically Pst, is the pressure that drives V̇max. It is informative to evaluate the relationship between V̇max and Pst. Figure 7-10A shows how this relationship is obtained, and Figure 7-10B shows its behavior in normal and diseased lungs.

In Figure 7-10A, flow–volume and static lung recoil curves for a healthy patient and a patient with pure emphysema are plotted on the common vertical axis of absolute lung volume. Thus, at any lung volume corresponding to the decreasing portion of the flow–volume curve, it is possible to measure simultaneous values of V̇max and Pst.

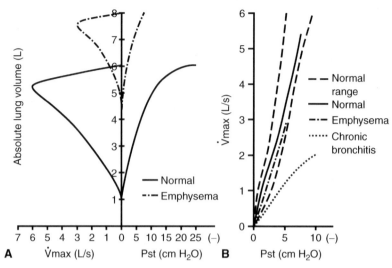

FIG. 7-10 **Relationships between maximal expiratory flow (V̇max) and lung static elastic recoil pressure (Pst).** A. V̇max and Pst are plotted on a common vertical absolute volume axis for a healthy patient and a patient with pure emphysema. B. Corresponding values of V̇max and Pst obtained at various lung volumes are plotted with V̇max as a function of Pst. This is called a maximal flow static recoil curve. In the case of chronic bronchitis, the flow–volume and Pst–volume curves are not shown. See text for further discussion.

In Figure 7-10B, Pst is plotted against V̇max at various lung volumes. Such a graph is called a maximal flow static recoil (MFSR) curve. The normal range of values is shown by the narrow space between the two dashed lines. Values obtained from the normal curve in Figure 7-10A are connected by the solid line. The same has been done for the case of pure emphysema. Because both the healthy patient and the patient with pure emphysema have no airway disease, the values fall within the normal range. This indicates that in the patient with emphysema, the decrease in maximal flow is caused mainly by the loss of lung recoil, not airways disease *per se*. However, if there is substantial chronic bronchitis, the MFSR curve is shifted down and to the right, indicating that, although there may be some loss of recoil pressure, this does not explain the decrease in flow, which is largely due to airway disease and the associated increase in airway resistance. The MFSR curve is useful in that it stresses the fact that V̇max may be reduced by either a loss of recoil pressure or substantial airway disease or both.

7E • Forced Oscillation Technique or Impulse Oscillometry System

This procedure was first described in 1956 and refined in the 1970s and 1980s but did not begin to be used clinically until 20 years ago because of improved instrumentation. The technique and its detailed explanation are complex. Basically, a large speaker is used to apply pressure/sound waves of various frequencies while the patient breathes quietly on the closed system. Small (~1 cm H_2O) oscillations of pressure are superimposed on the patient's breathing. The pressure, as reflected back from the lung, is used to calculate resistance at various frequencies as well as reactance, inertance, capacitance, and resonant frequency. Interpretation of these measurements is somewhat complex. The simplest to understand are the resistances at various frequencies. Measures at high frequencies (e.g., R20) are thought to reflect the proximal or large airways, whereas measures at low frequencies (R5) are thought to reflect airway total resistance. The difference between them (R5 − R20) is thought to reflect the small airways.[1] The potential advantages of the forced oscillation technique (FOT) or impulse oscillometry (IOS) are numerous. Both are noninvasive and can be used in infants and children, the elderly, and patients with cognitive or neuromuscular disabilities because no special breathing maneuvers are required. Both can also be used in sleep studies and in the intensive care unit. Both can be used to test for airway hyperreactivity. They do not require a deep inhalation, which can alter bronchomotor tone (see Case 32, pages 203-206), or forced expiratory maneuvers, which can be tiring and may alter bronchial tone. Despite these advantages, FOT or IOS has not been widely adopted and has been used mainly in infants and children younger than 5 years who are unable to perform spirometry or have difficulty with the procedure. Both have yet to be widely adopted in adult clinical medicine.

REFERENCE

1. Brashier B, Sundeep S. Measuring lung function using sound waves: role of the forced oscillation technique and impulse oscillometry system. *Breathe* 11:57–65, 2015.

chapter 8

Distribution of Ventilation

Various pathologic processes alter the normal pattern of ventilation distribution (i.e., the uniformity with which an inhaled breath is distributed to all the alveoli). For this reason, tests that detect abnormal patterns of ventilation distribution are fairly nonspecific and rarely of diagnostic importance. Their major contribution is that such abnormal patterns almost always are associated with alterations in ventilation–perfusion relationships (see pages 60 and 77). Abnormal distribution of ventilation also contributes to the frequency dependence of compliance (see page 77).

There are several tests of ventilation distribution. Some are complex and require sophisticated equipment and complex analysis. This chapter discusses only the simplest procedure, the single-breath nitrogen (SBN_2) test.

8A • Single-Breath Nitrogen Test

Procedure

The testing equipment and procedure are illustrated in Figure 8-1. The patient exhales to residual volume (RV) and then inhales a full breath of 100% oxygen from the bag on the left. A slow, complete exhalation

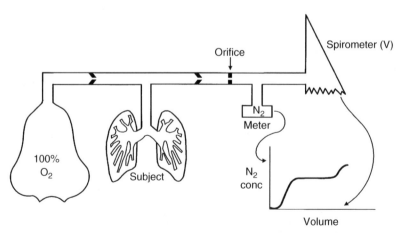

FIG. 8-1 Equipment required to perform the single-breath nitrogen washout test. A plot of exhaled nitrogen concentration (N_2 conc) against exhaled volume is shown at the lower right.

is directed by the one-way valve through the orifice past the nitrogen meter into the spirometer. The orifice ensures that expiratory flow will be steady and slow (<0.5 L/s), and we recommend its use. The nitrogen meter continuously records the nitrogen concentration of the expired gas as it enters the spirometer. With simultaneous plotting of the expired nitrogen concentration against expired volume, the normal graph shown in Figures 8-1 and 8-2A is obtained.

Normal Results

The plot in Figure 8-2A is from a seated normal patient. There are four important portions of the normal graph: phases I through IV.

To understand this graph, we need to consider how the inhaled oxygen is normally distributed in the lungs of a seated patient. At RV, the alveolar nitrogen concentration can be considered uniform (roughly 80%) throughout the lung, and alveolar gas is present in the trachea and upper airway (Fig. 8-3A). At RV, the alveoli (circles in Fig. 8-3A) in the more gravitationally dependent regions of the lung are at a smaller volume than those in the apical portions. Thus, the apical alveoli contain a larger volume of nitrogen at the same concentration. Therefore, as the patient inhales 100% oxygen, the apical alveoli receive proportionately less oxygen than the more dependent basal alveoli, and the alveolar nitrogen is less diluted than in the basal regions. Therefore, the nitrogen concentration is higher in the apical region. The result is a gradual decrease in nitrogen concentration farther down the lung, and the most

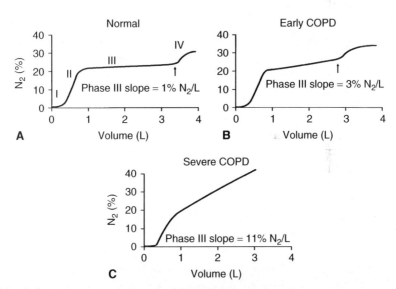

FIG. 8-2 Results of single-breath nitrogen washout tests on a normal patient (A), a patient with early chronic obstructive pulmonary disease (COPD) (B), and a patient with severe COPD (C). Closing volume (when present) is identified by an *arrow*. The various phases are identified on (A). The slope of phase III is given below each curve.

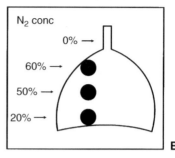

Residual Volume   Maximal Inspiration

A   B

FIG. 8-3 **Normal distribution of a breath of oxygen inhaled from residual volume and the resulting gravity-dependent alveolar nitrogen concentration (N_2 conc).** A. Lung at residual volume. B. Lung after a maximal inspiration to total lung capacity.

diluted alveolar gas is at the base (Fig. 8-3B). At the end of inspiration, the trachea and proximal airways contain only oxygen.

The events during expiration in the normal patient (Fig. 8-2A) are as follows. The initial gas passing the nitrogen meter comes from the trachea and upper airway and contains 100% oxygen. Thus, phase I shows 0% nitrogen. As expiration continues during phase II, alveolar gas begins washing out the dead space oxygen, and the nitrogen concentration gradually increases.

Phase III consists entirely of alveolar gas. During a slow expiration, initially, gas comes predominantly from the dependent alveolar regions, where the nitrogen concentration is lowest. As expiration continues, increasing amounts of gas come from the more apical regions, where nitrogen concentrations are higher. This sequence of events produces a gradually increasing nitrogen concentration during phase III. The normal slope of phase III is 1.0% to 2.5% nitrogen per liter expired. This value increases in the elderly.

An abrupt increase in nitrogen concentration occurs at the onset of phase IV. This reflects the decreased emptying of the dependent regions of the lung. Most of the final expiration comes from the apical regions, which have a higher concentration of nitrogen. The onset of phase IV is said to reflect the onset of airway closure in the dependent regions, and it is often called the closing volume. Whether airway closure actually occurs at this volume is debatable.[1] Normally, phase IV occurs with approximately 15% of the vital capacity still remaining. This value increases during normal aging, up to values of 25% of vital capacity.

8B • Changes in the Single-Breath Nitrogen Test in Disease

In obstructive lung disease, the SBN_2 test is altered in two ways (Fig. 8-2B). The lung volume at which phase IV occurs (closing volume) increases (less volume exhaled). In addition, the slope of phase III increases. This occurs because the normal pattern of gas distribution, including the vertical gradient of nitrogen concentration described previously, is gradually abolished. Disease occurs unevenly throughout the lung. Regions of greater disease with high airway flow resistance or high compliance empty less completely and hence receive less oxygen, and thus their nitrogen concentration is well above normal levels. Because the diseased areas empty more slowly than the more normal regions, the slope of phase III is greatly increased.

In more advanced obstructive disease (Fig. 8-2C), there is no longer a phase IV. It becomes lost in the very steep slope of phase III.

8C • Interpretation of the Single-Breath Nitrogen Test

The more nonuniform the distribution of ventilation, the steeper the slope of phase III. There are associated increases in the nonuniformity of the perfusion of the alveolar capillaries. The impact of these changes on arterial blood gases is noted in Section 6A, page 67.

It was thought that the increase in phase IV volume would be a useful, sensitive indicator of early airway disease. Unfortunately, it was not, and phase IV is rarely measured now. However, for many years phase III has been recognized as an excellent index of nonuniform ventilation. As shown in Figure 8-2, with the progress of obstructive airway disease, the slope of phase III progressively increases.

However, any measure of ventilation distribution is nonspecific. Increases in phase III are not limited to cases of airway obstruction. Increases also occur in pulmonary fibrosis, congestive heart failure, sarcoidosis, and other conditions in which airway disease is not the principal abnormality.

In conclusion, consideration of the distribution of ventilation tells much about lung physiology. Disorders of ventilation distribution are extremely important in the pathophysiology of conditions such as chronic bronchitis, asthma, and emphysema. In clinical practice, however, tests of ventilation distribution add very little to a basic battery of spirometry and tests of lung volumes, diffusing capacity, and arterial blood gases.

REFERENCE

1. Hyatt RE, Okeson GC, Rodarte JR. Influence of expiratory flow limitation on the pattern of lung emptying in normal man. *J Appl Physiol* 35:411–419, 1973.

chapter 9

Maximal Respiratory Pressures

In some clinical situations, evaluation of the strength of the respiratory muscles is very helpful. The strength of skeletal muscles, such as those of the arm, is easily tested by determining the force that they can develop, as by lifting weights. In contrast, the strength of the respiratory muscles can be determined by measuring the pressures developed against an occluded airway.

9A • Physiologic Principles

Some basic muscle physiology is reviewed here to aid in determining the best way of estimating the strength of respiratory muscles. Muscles, when maximally stimulated at different lengths, exhibit a characteristic length–tension behavior, as depicted in Figure 9-1. The greatest tension developed by the muscle occurs when it is at its optimal physiologic length. Less tension is developed at other lengths. To apply this concept to respiratory muscles, volume can be thought of as equivalent to length, and pressure as equivalent to tension. The *expiratory* muscles (chest wall and abdominal muscles) are at their optimal lengths near

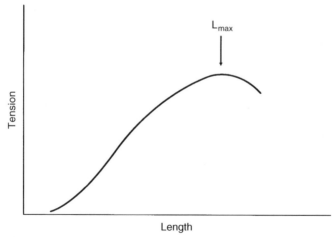

FIG. 9-1 Classic length–tension behavior of striated muscle. L_{max} is the length at which maximal tension can be developed.

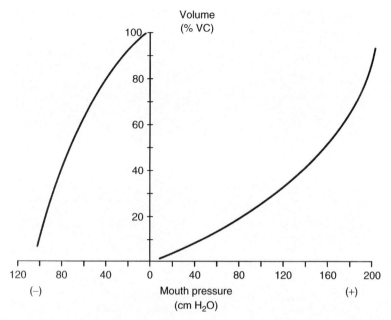

FIG. 9-2 **Maximal respiratory pressure that can be developed statically at various lung volumes (vital capacity [VC]).** Expiratory pressures are positive, and inspiratory pressures are negative. Total lung capacity is at 100% VC and residual volume at 0% VC.

total lung capacity. Figure 9-2 shows, as expected, that the highest expiratory pressures are generated near total lung capacity. The patient blows as hard as possible against an occluded airway. Conversely, near residual volume, the *inspiratory* muscles (primarily the diaphragm) are at their optimal lengths. Near residual volume, they develop the most negative pressure when the patient is sucking against an occluded airway. Therefore, the maximal strength of the expiratory muscles is measured near total lung capacity, and that of the inspiratory muscles is measured near residual volume.

9B • Measurement Techniques

The classic device used for these measurements is shown in Figure 9-3. It consists of a hollow stainless steel tube, to which are attached negative- and positive-pressure gauges. The distal end of the tube is occluded, except for a 2-mm hole. Modern equipment has electronic pressure transducers connected to computer processors. Function is the same but is less obvious on physical inspection.

Maximal expiratory pressure (PEmax) is measured as follows. The patient inhales maximally, holds the rubber tubing firmly against the mouth, and exhales as hard as possible. Several reproducible efforts are obtained, and the highest positive pressure maintained for a brief

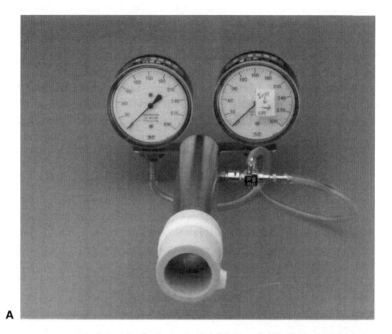

A

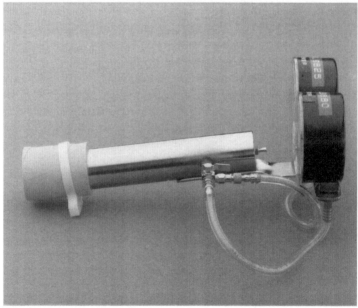

B

FIG. 9-3 Classic instrument used to measure maximal static expiratory and inspiratory pressures. The expiratory gauge measures 0 to +300 cm H_2O, and the inspiratory gauge 0 to −300 cm H_2O. Gauges are alternately connected to the cylinder by a three-way stopcock, as indicated by the *arrows* on the right-hand gauge (A). The side view (B) shows the small 2-mm hole at the distal end of the metal tube. A piece of firm rubber tubing is attached to the proximal end of the cylinder.

interval (usually 0.2–1.0 second) is recorded. Firm rubber tubing may be used rather than a standard cardboard or snorkel-type mouthpiece because at higher pressures (50–150 cm H_2O or more) air leaks around a conventional mouthpiece, the buccal muscles not being strong enough to maintain a tight seal. Such leaking is more common in patients with neuromuscular weakness. A nose clip is not usually required except for patients with muscle weakness.

Maximal inspiratory pressure (PImax) is measured by having the patient exhale to residual volume, hold the tubing against the lips, and suck as hard as possible. Again, the greatest negative pressure sustained for a similar interval is recorded. The small 2-mm hole at the distal end ensures that the device is measuring the pressure developed in the lung by the inspiratory muscles. Without it, if the patient closes the glottis and sucks with the cheeks, a very large negative pressure can be developed. The leak prevents this from happening because the pressure produced by sucking with a closed glottis decreases rapidly and cannot be sustained. To ensure accuracy, the patient must exert maximal effort. Herein lies a shortcoming of the test. These efforts can be uncomfortable. Some patients are unable, or unwilling, to make such effort. Enthusiastic coaching by the technician is essential.

9C • Normal Values

Normal values obtained from a motivated group of 60 healthy male and 60 healthy female patients are listed in Table 9-1. As Figure 9-2 shows, PEmax is roughly double the PImax. Male patients developed greater pressures than female patients, and in both sexes pressure declined with age, except for inspiratory pressures in male patients.

TABLE 9-1 **Normal Values for Maximal Respiratory Pressures, by Age**					
			Age (years)		
Pressure	20–54	55–59	60–64	65–69	70–74
PImax, cm H_2O[a]					
Male	-124 ± 44	-103 ± 32	-103 ± 32	-103 ± 32	-103 ± 32
Female	-87 ± 32	-77 ± 26	-73 ± 26	-70 ± 26	-65 ± 26
PEmax, cm H_2O[a]					
Male	233 ± 84	218 ± 74	209 ± 74	197 ± 74	185 ± 74
Female	152 ± 54	145 ± 40	140 ± 40	135 ± 40	128 ± 40

[a]Numbers represent mean ± 2 standard deviations.
PEmax, maximal expiratory pressure; PImax, maximal inspiratory pressure.

9D • Indications for Maximal Respiratory Pressure Measurements

1. In patients with neuromuscular disease who have dyspnea, measurement of respiratory muscle strength is a more sensitive test than spirometry or maximal voluntary ventilation.[1] We studied 10 patients with early neuromuscular diseases (amyotrophic lateral sclerosis, myasthenia gravis, and polymyositis). Eight of the 10 had considerable dyspnea, but only 2 had a significant reduction in vital capacity (77%). Five had a reduced maximal voluntary ventilation (73%). However, nine patients had significant reductions in $P_{E}max$ (47% predicted) and $P_{I}max$ (34% predicted). In the early stages, dyspnea was best explained by a reduction in respiratory muscle strength at a time when the strength of other skeletal muscles was little impaired. Table 9-2 lists some neuromuscular conditions in which respiratory muscle weakness has been encountered.

2. It is useful to measure respiratory muscle strength in the cooperative patient with an isolated, unexplained decrease in the vital capacity or maximal voluntary ventilation. Such decreases could be early signs of respiratory muscle weakness and could explain a complaint of dyspnea. Other conditions in which muscle weakness has been documented are lupus erythematosus, lead poisoning, scleroderma, and hyperthyroidism.

PEARL An effective cough is generally not possible when maximal expiratory pressure is less than 40 cm H_2O.

Unexplained fainting may be caused by cough syncope in the patient with severe chronic bronchitis. Sustained airway pressures of more than 300 cm H_2O have been measured in this condition during paroxysms of coughing. Such pressures are sufficient to reduce venous return and thus cardiac output, leading to syncope, occasionally even when the patient is supine.

TABLE 9-2 **Neuromuscular Disorders Associated with Respiratory Muscle Weakness**

Amyotrophic lateral sclerosis	Guillain–Barré syndrome
Myasthenia gravis	Syringomyelia
Muscular dystrophy	Parkinson disease
Polymyositis, dermatomyositis	Steroid myopathy
Poliomyelitis, postpolio syndrome	Polyneuropathy
Stroke	Spinal cord injury
Diaphragm paralysis	Acid maltase deficiency

3. Measurement of respiratory muscle strength in the intensive care unit has been used as an assessment of readiness to wean from mechanical ventilation. A pressure transducer can be connected to the 15-mm adapter on the endotracheal tube. If testing is performed for patients who are not intubated (as a measure of risk of respiratory failure in patients with respiratory muscle weakness), it is important to have the small leak in the device, as described in Section 9B.

When maximal respiratory pressures are used for assessment of weaning potential, inspiratory pressure greater than -20 to 30 cm H_2O and expiratory pressure greater than $+30$ to 50 cm H_2O have been identified to be predictive of the ability to wean patients from ventilatory support. However, the use of a single factor in deciding about weaning potential is not encouraged. It must be kept in mind that the ability to breathe unassisted depends on the balance between the capacity of the respiratory muscles to perform work and the workload imposed on the respiratory muscles by the chest wall and lungs.

REFERENCE

1. Black LF, Hyatt RE. Maximal static respiratory pressures in generalized neuromuscular disease. *Am Rev Respir Dis* 103:641–650, 1971.

chapter 10

Preoperative Pulmonary Function Testing

The goals of preoperative pulmonary function testing are (1) to detect unrecognized lung disease, (2) to estimate the risk of operation compared with the potential benefit, (3) to plan perioperative care, and (4) to estimate postoperative lung function. Several studies have shown a high prevalence of unsuspected impairment of lung function in surgical patients and suggest that preoperative pulmonary function testing is underused. There is evidence that appropriate perioperative management improves surgical outcome in patients with impaired lung function.

10A • Who Should Be Tested?

The indications for testing depend on the characteristics of the patient and on the planned surgical procedure. Table 10-1 lists the characteristics of the patient and the surgical procedures for which testing is

TABLE 10-1 **Indications for Preoperative Pulmonary Function Testing**
Patient
Known pulmonary dysfunction
Currently smoking, especially if >1 pack per day
Chronic productive cough
Recent respiratory infection
Advanced age
Obesity >30% over ideal weight
Thoracic cage deformity, such as kyphoscoliosis
Neuromuscular disease, such as amyotrophic lateral sclerosis or myasthenia gravis
Procedure
Thoracic or upper abdominal operation
Pulmonary resection
Prolonged anesthesia

recommended. We believe that preoperative testing should be done on all patients scheduled for any lung resection. We also recommend testing before upper abdominal and thoracic operation in patients with known lung disease and for smokers older than 40 years (up to one-fourth of such smokers have abnormal lung function) because these procedures present the greatest risk for patients with impaired lung function. When a significant abnormality is detected, appropriate perioperative intervention may reduce the morbidity and mortality related to operation. Such intervention includes the use of bronchodilators and postoperative use of incentive spirometry. Although the benefit of smoking cessation before operation has not been proved, it is common practice to recommend that smokers, especially those with impaired lung function, stop smoking several weeks before surgery.

10B • What Tests Should Be Done?

For patients with obstructive disorders, spirometry before and after bronchodilator therapy may be sufficient preoperative testing. However, for those with moderate-to-severe airway obstruction, arterial carbon dioxide tension (blood gases) should also be measured. Table 10-2 lists general guidelines for interpreting test results in terms of risk to the patient.

The risk of surgical procedures for patients with restrictive disorders is less well studied than that for patients with obstructive disorders. We recommend following similar guidelines but keeping in mind the cause of restriction (parenchymal lung disease, chest wall disorders, muscle weakness, and obesity).

Indications for measurement of the diffusing capacity of the lungs (DLCO) are not clearly established. We recommend that DLCO be measured in patients with restrictive disorders to evaluate the severity of gas exchange abnormality. In pulmonary parenchymal disorders, such as pulmonary fibrosis, this abnormality is often more severe than expected from the degree of ventilatory impairment alone.

TABLE 10-2 Guidelines for Estimating the Risk of Postoperative Respiratory Complications

Test	Increased Risk	High Risk
FVC	<50% predicted	≤1.5 L
FEV_1	<2.0 L or <50% predicted	<1.0 L
MVV		<50% predicted
$Paco_2$		≥45 mm Hg

FEV_1, forced expiratory volume in 1 second; FVC, forced expiratory vital capacity; MVV, maximal voluntary ventilation; $Paco_2$, arterial carbon dioxide tension.

Oximetry is an inexpensive measure of gas exchange but is relatively nonspecific and insensitive, even when performed during exercise. We do not recommend its use for determining operative risk. It is useful, however, for monitoring oxygen therapy postoperatively.

Maximal voluntary ventilation is also used as a predictor of postoperative respiratory complications. It is less reproducible than forced expiratory volume in 1 second (FEV_1) and is more dependent on muscle strength and effort. For these reasons, it is no longer used to determine a patient's eligibility for Social Security disability payments. However, it does have a role in preoperative assessment and is comparable to FEV_1 for predicting postoperative respiratory complications. We also find it useful as an indicator of respiratory muscle strength.

10C • Additional Studies

Quantitative radionuclide scintigraphy has been used to determine regional ventilation and perfusion of the lungs. The results have been used to improve estimates of postoperative pulmonary function, especially for patients with marginal lung function.

Maximal cardiopulmonary exercise studies have been used for preoperative assessment. Several authors have reported low rates of postoperative complications in patients with a maximal oxygen uptake of more than 20 mL/kg/min and high rates of complications with a maximal oxygen uptake of less than 15 mL/kg/min. This form of testing requires sophisticated equipment and considerable technical expertise. It is therefore more expensive than other tests. Yet the cost of testing is small compared with that of most surgical procedures.

10D • What Is Prohibitive Risk?

Several algorithms have been developed for calculation of lung function after resection of lung tissue. One approach requires an estimation of the number of lung segments, out of a total of 18, that are likely to be removed. Then the following calculation is performed:

$$\text{Preoperative } FEV_1 \times \frac{\text{(No. of remaining segments)}}{18} = \text{Postoperative } FEV_1 \qquad \text{(Eq. 1)}$$

Thus, if five segments are to be removed and the preoperative FEV_1 is 2.0 L, the predicted postoperative FEV_1 is 1.4 L:

$$\left(2 \times \frac{18-5}{18}\right) = 1.4$$

Postoperative FEV_1 predicted from this calculation is the estimated level of lung function after full recovery, not immediately after operation. In the past, a common recommendation was that surgical resection should not be performed if the predicted postoperative FEV_1 was less than 0.8 L. However, several studies show that with modern postoperative care, this is no longer an absolute contraindication. Specialized centers with excellent perioperative care have reported low morbidity and mortality in such severely impaired patients.[1]

REFERENCE

1. Cerfolio RJ, Allen MS, Trastek VF, Deschamps C, Scanlon PD, Pairolero PC. Lung resection in patients with compromised pulmonary function. *Ann Thorac Surg* 62:348–351, 1996.

chapter 11

Simple Tests of Exercise Capacity

In most instances, the clinician has an estimate of a patient's exercise capacity. This is based on the history, results of physical examination, and pertinent data, such as chest radiographs, electrocardiogram, blood cell count, and standard pulmonary function tests, possibly including arterial blood gas values.

However, in some situations, a quantitative estimate of a patient's exercise capacity is needed. Before formal exercise studies are requested, some relatively simple tests can be performed. These can be done in the office or in a hospital's pulmonary function laboratory. They may obviate more extensive testing by providing a sufficient assessment of a patient's limitation.

11A • Exercise Oximetry

Pulse oximetry, available in most hospitals, is an inexpensive and noninvasive method of estimating arterial oxygen saturation in the absence of high concentrations of abnormal hemoglobins. After an appropriate site for exercising is selected and pulse oximetry quality assurance criteria are satisfied, oxygen saturation at rest is recorded. If resting saturation is normal or near normal, the patient exercises until he or she is short of breath. In some disease entities, such as pulmonary fibrosis, pulmonary hypertension, and emphysema, values at rest are normal, but surprising desaturation is noted with exercise. In this situation, a wise step is to repeat the exercise with the patient breathing oxygen to determine whether the saturation is easily corrected and the dyspnea ameliorated.

If a patient's resting saturation is low, this may be all the information needed. If supplemental oxygen is to be prescribed, however, the flow rates of oxygen that will provide adequate resting and mild exertion saturation may need to be determined.

For such studies, it is important to record the distance and time walked. For prescribing oxygen, the levels of exercise (distance walked) can be compared without and with supplemental oxygen. In some patients with chronic obstructive pulmonary disease (COPD) and those with chest wall and neuromuscular limitations in whom carbon dioxide retention may be of concern, resting arterial blood gas values while the patient is breathing the prescribed oxygen concentration should be obtained to rule out progressive hypercapnia. Determining arterial blood gas values during exercise while breathing the prescribed oxygen concentration is generally not necessary.

> **PEARL** • In a few situations, the saturation is falsely low when the pulse oximeter is used on the finger. These situations include thick calluses, excessive ambient light, use of dark shades of nail polish, jaundice, and conditions with poor peripheral circulation such as scleroderma and Raynaud disease. In cases with a poor pulse signal, the earlobe or forehead is an alternative site. If there is any doubt about the reliability of the oximeter readings, or if the reading does not match the clinical situation, arterial blood gas studies are recommended.

11B • 6-Minute Walk Tests

Simple walking tests are useful for quantifying and documenting a patient's exercise capacity over time. They can be used in both pulmonary and cardiac diseases with reasonable precautions. They are also valuable for quantifying the progress of patients in rehabilitation programs. The relative merits of the 6-minute walk test (6MWT) versus the cardiopulmonary exercise test and shuttle-walk test are debated. The 6MWT has become the predominant standard and is the best-studied and best-characterized simple exercise test.[1]

The test is best performed in an unobstructed level corridor, preferably 100 ft or 30 m in length, with minimal competing traffic. The patient is instructed to walk back and forth over the course and go as far as possible in 6 minutes. The patient should be encouraged by standardized statements such as "You're doing well" and "Keep up the good work." Patients are allowed to stop and rest during the test but are encouraged to resume walking as soon as possible. The number of laps is counted and additional distance measured for total distance walked. Pulse rate is recorded before and after the test or can be monitored in real time. If the patient is using oxygen, the flow rate and mode of transport, such as carried or pulled unit, are recorded. The report should include distance walked rounded to the nearest foot or meter. It can be reported as a percentage of the reference value from a standard reference. The report may also include the average speed, number and duration of stops, baseline and minimum saturation, baseline and maximum or end-of-test heart rate, and symptoms. Table 11-1 relates the distances walked to the average rate of walking in miles per hour. Prediction equations for the 6MWT are available for average healthy adults 40 to 80 years old.[2] These are listed in Table 11-1. The use of the test is twofold. First, by comparing a patient's results with the predicted norm, the patient's degree of impairment can be estimated. Second, the test is most valuable as a measure of the patient's response to therapy or the progression of disease.

11C • Stair-Climbing Test

For many years, physicians have used stair climbing to estimate a patient's cardiopulmonary reserve. The empirical nature of stair climbing has been a drawback. However, in one study, subjects with COPD climbed stairs

TABLE 11-1	**Relation of 6- and 12-Minute Walks to Speed**	
	Distance (ft) Walked In	
Speed (mph)	**6 min**	**12 min**
3	1,584	3,168
2	1,056	2,112
1	528	1,056
0.5	264	528
0.25	132	264

Prediction equations for the distance walked during the 6-minute walk test (6MWD) for adults 40 to 80 years old. Results are given in meters (1 m = 3.28 ft).[2] Men: 6MWD = (7.57 × height in cm) − (5.02 × age in years) − (1.76 × weight in kg) − 309 m. Women: 6MWD = (2.11 × height in cm) − (5.78 × age in years) − (2.29 × weight in kg) + 667 m.[2]

until they became limited by symptoms and stopped.[3] A significant correlation was found between the number of steps climbed and (1) peak oxygen consumption ($\dot{V}O_2$) and (2) maximal exercise ventilation ($\dot{V}E$). This test is another way to estimate operative risk in patients with COPD who are to undergo thoracic operation. The study found that, on average, the ability to climb 83 steps was equivalent to a maximal $\dot{V}O_2$ ($\dot{V}O_2$max) of 20 mL/kg/min. The ability to reach a $\dot{V}O_2$max of 20 mL/kg/min has been reported to be associated with fewer complications after lung resection or thoracotomy.

Stair climbing is more cumbersome than the 6MWT or 12-minute walk. However, it does push most patients closer to their $\dot{V}O_2$max, an end point of greater physiologic significance.

11D • Ventilatory Reserve

Measuring a patient's ventilation during a given task or exercise provides an estimate of the demand of that task. The definition of ventilatory reserve (VR) is given by this relationship:

$$VR = \frac{MVV - exercise\ ventilation(\dot{V}E)}{MVV} \times 100 \quad (Eq.\ 1)$$

Given a maximal voluntary ventilation (MVV) of 60 L/min and $\dot{V}E$ of 30 L/min during a given task, the VR is 50% ([60–30]/60). The greater the $\dot{V}E$, the lower the reserve, and the more likely it is that the patient will become dyspneic. A VR of less than 50% is usually associated with dyspnea. Another approach is to subtract $\dot{V}E$ from the MVV. A value of MVV − $\dot{V}E$ less than 20 L/min indicates severe ventilatory limitation.

11E • Rating of Respiratory Impairment Using Pulmonary Function Tests

The most common approach to estimating respiratory impairment is based on the percentage reduction in various pulmonary function tests. A recommendation presented by the American Thoracic Society (ATS)

TABLE 11-2 **Estimations of Respiratory Impairment Based on Results of Pulmonary Function Tests**

Condition	Test[a]				
	FVC	FEV$_1$	FEV$_1$/FVC	D$_{LCO}$	$\dot{V}_{O_2}$max
Normal	>80	>80	>75	>80	>75
Mild impairment	60–80	60–80	60–75	60–80	60–75
Moderate impairment (unable to meet physical requirements of many jobs)	50–60	40–60	40–60	40–60	40–60
Severe impairment (unable to meet most job demands, including travel to work)	<50	<40	<40	<40	<40

[a]All tests relate to the percentage of the normal predicted value for an individual.
D$_{LCO}$, diffusing capacity of carbon monoxide; FEV$_1$, forced expiratory volume in 1 second; FVC, forced expiratory vital capacity; $\dot{V}_{O_2}$max, maximal oxygen consumption.
Data from American Thoracic Society Ad Hoc Committee on Impairment/Disability Evaluation. Evaluation of impairment/disability secondary to respiratory disorders. *Am Rev Respir Dis* 133:1205–1209, 1986. Used with permission.

in 1986 is summarized in Table 11-2.[4] It provides useful guidelines. The recommendation was revised in 2005 by the ATS in conjunction with the European Respiratory Society (ERS).[5] It is controversial, and our laboratory does not follow the recent recommendations.[6] Laboratory directors should evaluate such recommendations critically.

If a patient complains of severe dyspnea but the tests show only mild-to-moderate impairment, muscle weakness, upper airway obstruction, or causes other than respiratory should be considered. If none are found, cardiopulmonary exercise testing is often helpful to define the cause of exercise limitation.

11F • Cardiopulmonary Exercise Testing

Cardiopulmonary exercise testing requires sophisticated equipment and should be performed only by laboratories with strict quality control, experienced physiologic direction, appropriate medical supervision, and considerable experience in doing such tests.[7] Numerous variables of gas exchange and cardiac function, some requiring an indwelling arterial catheter for repeated blood gas determinations, are measured. The measurements include minute ventilation ($\dot{V}_E$), oxygen consumption ($\dot{V}_{O_2}$), carbon dioxide production ($\dot{V}_{CO_2}$), dead space ventilation, and alveolar–arterial oxygen gradients. In some laboratories, $\dot{V}_{O_2}$ and $\dot{V}_{CO_2}$ are measured breath by breath. Also measured are the heart rate, blood pressure, and lactate levels, and electrocardiography is performed.

Some of the indications for cardiopulmonary exercise testing are as follows:

■ To distinguish between cardiac and pulmonary causes of dyspnea in complex cases

■ To determine whether the patient's symptoms are caused by deconditioning
■ To detect the malingering patient
■ To provide disability evaluation in problem cases
■ To determine the level of fitness, including whether a patient can meet the work requirements of a given work assignment

REFERENCES

1. Holland AE, Spruit MA, Troosters T, et al. An official European Respiratory Society/American Thoracic Society technical standard: field walking tests in chronic respiratory disease. *Eur Respir J* 44:1428–1446, 2014. doi:10.1183/09031936.00150314.
2. Enright PL, Sherrill DL. Reference equations for the six-minute walk in healthy adults. *Am J Respir Crit Care Med* 158:1384–1387, 1998.
3. Pollock M, Roa J, Benditt J, Celli B. Estimation of ventilatory reserve by stair climbing: a study in patients with chronic airflow obstruction. *Chest* 104:1378–1383, 1993.
4. American Thoracic Society Ad Hoc Committee on Impairment/Disability Evaluation. Evaluation of impairment/disability secondary to respiratory disorders. *Am Rev Respir Dis* 133:1205–1209, 1986.
5. Pellegrino R, Viegi G, Brusasco V, et al. Interpretative strategies for lung function tests. *Eur Respir J* 26:948–968, 2005. doi:10.1183/09031936.05.00035205.
6. Enright PL. Flawed interpretative strategies for lung function tests harm patients. *Eur Respir J* 27(6):1322–1323, 2006.
7. Jones NL, Killian KJ. Exercise limitation in health and disease. *N Engl J Med* 343:632–641, 2000.

chapter 12

Patterns in Various Diseases

There are patterns of pulmonary function test abnormalities that are typical for most patients with a particular disease. Table 12-1 expands on Table 3-1, adding data on lung volumes, arterial blood gas values, diffusing capacity, lung compliance and resistance, the single-breath nitrogen test, and maximal respiratory pressures. It should be emphasized that a clinical diagnosis is not made from these test results alone; rather they quantify the lung impairment and are to be interpreted in the context of the total clinical picture. For this discussion, obstructive disease is categorized into four conditions: emphysema, chronic bronchitis, chronic obstructive pulmonary disease, and asthma. Restrictive conditions are divided into those due to pulmonary parenchymal disease and extrapulmonary causes.

12A • Emphysema

Pure emphysema (such as α_1-antitrypsin deficiency) is associated with hyperinflation (increased total lung capacity [TLC]); a significant loss of lung elasticity (decreased recoil pressure at TLC and increased static compliance of the lung [PTLC and $C_{L_{stat}}$]); and often a substantial decrease in the diffusing capacity of the lung (DLCO, reflecting destruction of alveoli). Resting arterial tension of oxygen (PaO$_2$) and carbon dioxide (PaCO$_2$) are generally normal until the condition is far advanced. Bullae, predominantly in the lower lung fields, are typical in α_1-antitrypsin deficiency.

12B • Chronic Bronchitis

Pure chronic bronchitis is typically found in heavy cigarette smokers with a chronic productive cough and frequent respiratory infections. In contrast to emphysema, lung recoil is often normal, but the PaO$_2$ may be low and associated with carbon dioxide retention (increased PaCO$_2$).

12C • Chronic Obstructive Pulmonary Disease

The lungs of most smokers in whom obstructive lung disease develops show a mixture of emphysema and chronic bronchitis. The tests reflect

Table 12-1 Patterns of Pulmonary Function Tests in Disease

Test	Units	Emphysema	Chronic Bronchitis	Chronic Obstructive Pulmonary Disease	Asthma	Restrictive Intrapulmonary	Restrictive Extrapulmonary	Neuromuscular Disease	Congestive Heart Failure	Obesity
FVC	L	(N)→↓	(N)→↓	(N)→↓	↓	↓	↓	N→↓	↓	N→↓
FEV$_1$	L	↓	↓	↓	↓	↓	↓	N→↓	↓	N→↓
FEV$_1$/FVC	%	↓	↓	↓	N→↓	N→↑	N	N	N→↓	N
FEF$_{25-75}$	L/s	↓	↓	↓	↓	N→↓	↓	N→↓	↓	N→↓
PEF	L/min	↓	↓	↓	↓	N→↓	↓	N→↓	↓	N
MW	L/min	↓	↓	↓	↓	N→↓	↓	N→↓	↓	N→↓
FEF$_{50}$	L/s	↓	↓	–	↓	N→↓	↓	N→↓	↓	N→↓
Slope of FV curve		↓	↓	–	N→↑	↑	N→↑	N	N→↑	N
TLC	L	↑	N→↑	↑	N	↓	↓	N→↑	↓	N→↑
RV	L	↑	↑	↑	↑	↓	↓	N→↑	N→↑	N→↑→↓
RV/TLC	%	↑	↑	↑	↑	N	N→↑	N→↑	N→↑	N→↑
DLco	mL/mm Hg/min	↓	N→↓	N→↓	↓N↑→↑	↓	N	N→↑	↓	N
DL/VA	mL/mm Hg/min/L	↓	N→↑	N→↑	↓N↑→↑	↓→N	N	N	↓	N→↑
Pao$_2$	torr[a]	N→↓	↓	N→↓	N→↓	↓	N	N→↓	N→↓	N→↓

98

Sao$_2$	%	N→↓	N	N	→	N	N	N	N→↑
Paco$_2$	torr[a]	N→←	N	N	N→←	N	N	N	N→↑
pH	−log[H⁺]	N→↑	N	N→↑	N→↑	N	N	N	N→↑
Raw	cm H$_2$O/L/s	←	↓N↑↑	←	↑	N→↑	N→↑	N→↑	N→↑
Cl$_{stat}$	L/cm H$_2$O	←	N→↑	N	N→↑	N	N	N	N→↑
Cl$_{dyn}$	L/cm H$_2$O	←	N→↑	→	N→↑	N	N	N	N→↑
PTLC	cm H$_2$O	←	→	N→←	N	N	N	N	N→↑
Phase III	% N$_2$/L	←	←	N→←	←	N	N	N	N→←
Phase IV	% vital capacity	A	↑→A	↑→A	N→↑	N	N	N	N→↑
Pemax	cm H$_2$O	←	↓→N→↑	N	N→↑	N	N	N	N→↓↓
Pimax	cm H$_2$O	↓	N→↑	N→↑	N→↑	N	N	N	N→↓↓

[a]torr, equivalent to mm Hg.

→, to; ↑, increased; ↓, decreased; A, often absent; Cl$_{dyn}$, dynamic compliance of the lung; Cl$_{stat}$, static compliance of the lung; Dlco, diffusing capacity of carbon monoxide; DL/VA, diffusing capacity of the lung/alveolar volume; FEF$_{25-75}$, forced expiratory flow rate over the middle 50% of the FVC; FEF$_{50}$, forced expiratory flow after 50% of the FVC has been exhaled; FEV$_1$, forced expiratory volume in 1 second; FV, flow-volume; FVC, forced vital capacity; MVV, maximal voluntary ventilation; N, normal; (N), occasionally normal; Paco$_2$, arterial carbon dioxide tension; Pao$_2$, arterial oxygen tension; PEF, peak expiratory flow; Pemax, maximal expiratory pressure; Pimax, maximal inspiratory pressure; PTLC, lung recoil pressure at TLC; Raw, airway resistance; RV, residual volume; Sao$_2$, arterial oxygen saturation; TLC, total lung capacity.

contributions of both disease processes. For example, hyperinflation tends to be greater than in pure chronic bronchitis, but carbon dioxide retention may not be present.

12D • Asthma

Because lung function may be normal between attacks, the data in Table 12-1 reflect those during a moderate asthma exacerbation in a nonsmoker. The changes are much like those in chronic obstructive pulmonary disease, except for the tendency toward hyperventilation and respiratory alkalosis (increased pH and decreased $Paco_2$). In addition, the response to bronchodilators (not shown in Table 12-1) is typically very striking and DLCO is often increased. In remission, all test results, with the occasional exception of the residual volume/TLC ratio (RV/TLC), may return to normal; however, the methacholine challenge test is typically positive. The ratio of forced expiratory volume in 1 second to forced expiratory vital capacity (FEV_1/FVC) may be normal, especially in mild cases. The DLCO may be normal or increased. It is decreased only in very severe asthma.

12E • Pulmonary Restriction

Idiopathic pulmonary fibrosis is the classic example of a pulmonary parenchymal restrictive process. Lung volumes are reduced, expiratory flows may be normal or low, the diffusion capacity decreased, PTLC generally increased, lung compliance decreased, and the slope of the expiratory flow–volume (FV) curve steep.

Some other parenchymal conditions that cause restriction are listed in Table 12-2. However, not all of them always produce the classic picture described here. The slope of the FV curve may not be increased and the lung recoil may not be altered, in part because varying degrees of restriction may be combined with varying degrees of obstruction. Examples are endobronchial involvement in sarcoidosis and tuberculosis. This mixed pattern is also frequent in heart failure, cystic fibrosis, and Langerhans' cell histiocytosis (eosinophilic granuloma or histiocytosis X) and lymphangioleiomyomatosis.

12F • Extrapulmonary Restriction

In cases of extrapulmonary restriction, the lung parenchyma is typically normal. The most frequent causes of this type of restriction are listed in Table 12-2. The main abnormalities are the decreased lung volumes with generally normal gas exchange. Because the DLCO is somewhat volume dependent, it may be reduced. Resection in an otherwise normal lung also fits this pattern.

Severe degrees of restriction, as in advanced kyphoscoliosis, can lead to respiratory insufficiency with abnormal gas exchange.

TABLE 12-2 **Causes of Restrictive Disease**
Pulmonary
Pulmonary fibrosis and interstitial pneumonitis
Asbestosis
Neoplasms, including lymphangitic carcinoma
Pneumonia
Sarcoidosis (Stage 3)
Bronchiolitis obliterans with organizing pneumonia or cryptogenic organizing pneumonia
Hypersensitivity pneumonitis
Pulmonary alveolar proteinosis
Langerhans' cell histiocytosis (histiocytosis X or eosinophilic granuloma)
Lung resection
Atelectasis
Extrapulmonary
Pleural cavity
Pleural effusion
Pneumothorax
Fibrothorax
Cardiac enlargement
Neuromuscular
Diaphragmatic paralysis
Neuromuscular diseases (see Table 9-2)
Chest wall
Obesity
Kyphoscoliosis
Ankylosing spondylitis
Chest trauma
Thoracic resection
Abdominal mass (pregnancy, ascites, bulky tumor)

12G • Neuromuscular Disease

The hallmark of early neuromuscular disease is a decrease in respiratory muscle strength reflected by decreases in maximal expiratory and inspiratory pressures. At this stage, all other test results can be normal despite the patient complaining of exertional dyspnea. As the process progresses, the maximal voluntary ventilation decreases next, followed by the FVC and TLC with accompanying impairment of gas exchange. Ultimately, the picture fits that of a restrictive extrapulmonary disorder.

These progressive patterns are most frequently observed in amyotrophic lateral sclerosis, myasthenia gravis, and polymyositis. They have also been noted in syringomyelia, muscular dystrophy, parkinsonism, various myopathies, and Guillain–Barré syndrome.

12H • Congestive Heart Failure

The effects of left-sided congestive heart failure with pulmonary congestion on the function of an otherwise normal lung are often not appreciated. In some cases, the predominant change is one of pure restriction with a normal FEV_1/FVC ratio, flows decreased in proportion to the FVC, and a normal FV curve slope. There is often associated cardiomegaly or pleural effusion, which contribute to restriction. The chest radiograph may be interpreted as suggesting interstitial fibrosis, but the computed tomographic appearance is distinctly different.

In other cases, there may be a mixed restrictive–obstructive pattern, or pure obstruction, with decreases in flow out of proportion to volume reduction. The FEV_1/FVC ratio is reduced, as is the slope of the FV curve. The obstructive component is in part caused by peribronchial edema, which narrows the airways and produces "cardiac asthma." Of interest, the result of the methacholine challenge test may be positive for reasons that are unclear.

In years past, the effectiveness of therapy for pulmonary congestion was sometimes monitored by measuring changes in the vital capacity. Congestive heart failure is highlighted here because it is often overlooked as a possible cause of a restrictive or obstructive pattern.

12I • Obesity

The changes in pulmonary function tests associated with obesity are indicated in Table 12-1.[1] These changes do not seem to differ substantially between male and female patients. Some test results, such as the TLC, are abnormal only in patients with a very high body mass index. Others, such as decreases in functional residual capacity and expiratory reserve volume (particularly the latter, which is not included in Table 12-1), occur with milder degrees of obesity. The results for RV and RV/TLC ratio may depend in part on whether the RV was calculated using the FVC or slow vital capacity (see Section 3C, page 26). Even in very obese patients, the FEV_1/FVC ratio is typically normal. The effects of obesity on pulmonary function are greater in patients with a truncal fat distribution ("apple" vs. "pear") and may be greater in the elderly and in smokers, variables that are not always reported. In this respect, one study[2] found that male patients who had obstructive lung disease and gained weight after quitting smoking had a loss of 17.4 mL in FVC for every kilogram of weight gained. Their FEV_1 also decreased by 11.1 mL/kg of weight gained. Similar but smaller losses of 10.6 mL from FVC and 5.6 mL from FEV_1 were observed in women.

An interesting question has arisen with the association between obesity and asthma. Does obesity cause asthma? The final answer is not in. One review[3] concluded that obesity has an important but modest impact on the incidence and prevalence of asthma. More recently, obesity has been increasingly recognized as a major risk factor for asthma in adults and children. Obese asthmatics seem to have a distinct phenotype. The mechanisms behind the association between obesity and asthma are the subject of considerable research.[4]

REFERENCES

1. Jones RL, Nzekwu MM. The effects of body mass index on lung volumes. *Chest* 130:827–833, 2006.
2. Wise RA, Enright PL, Connett JE, et al. Effect of weight gain on pulmonary function after smoking cessation in the Lung Health Study. *Am J Respir Crit Care Med* 157:866–872, 1998.
3. Beuther DA, Weiss ST, Sutherland ER. Obesity and asthma. *Am J Respir Crit Care Med* 174:112–119, 2006.
4. Peters U, Dixon AE, Forno E. Obesity and asthma. *J Allerg Clin Immunol* 141:1169–1179, 2018.

chapter 13

When to Test and
What to Order

The recommendations for *preoperative* testing are listed in Chapter 10. Although there are many other situations in which pulmonary function testing is indicated, for reasons that are unclear these tests are underutilized. Among patients with a diagnosis of chronic obstructive pulmonary disease (COPD), a large proportion have not been tested, and among the untested, a large proportion do not have obstruction and are, hence, incorrectly overdiagnosed. There are also many who are untested and have undiagnosed COPD. This chapter describes instances in which testing is warranted and includes the basic tests to be ordered. Depending on the initial test results, additional studies may be indicated.

13A • The Smoker

Some advocates have argued that all current and former smokers should have screening spirometry regardless of symptoms. In order to defend that recommendation, we would need a controlled trial showing that screening spirometry improves the rate of smoking cessation among young smokers. Such studies have not been done. It is worth noting that 50% to 75% of smokers do not develop COPD. This means that normal results from screening spirometry could even encourage smokers with normal spirometry to believe they are spared of adverse effects and to continue smoking. The U.S. Preventive Services Task Force noted that: "Spirometry has not been shown to independently increase smoking cessation rates. . . . No direct evidence indicates that screening patients for COPD using spirometry improves long-term health outcomes."[1]

On the other hand, adult smokers with symptoms of obstruction should be tested with spirometry at virtually any age. Smokers develop the earliest adverse effects of smoking on lung function in their 20s by not reaching their full growth of lung function. After that, there is normally a plateau in lung function between ages 20 to 25 and 35 to 40, but in susceptible smokers, lung function begins to decline in the 20s. After the age of 35, the rate of decline in forced expiratory volume in 1 second (FEV_1) and forced expiratory vital capacity (FVC), normally about 30 mL/y, doubles to about 60 mL/y in susceptible smokers.[2] In the Lung Health study, smokers with COPD were identified as early as 35 years of age.

Depending on the results of spirometry and a patient's smoking habits, repeat testing every 3 to 5 years may be reasonable. The logic for

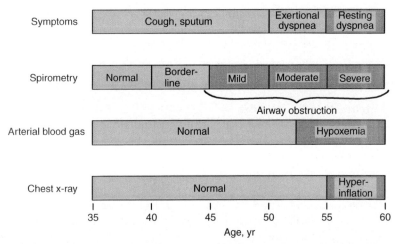

FIG. 13-1 **Progression of symptoms in chronic obstructive pulmonary disease (COPD) reflected by spirometry, arterial blood gas studies, and chest radiographs as a function of age in a typical case.** Spirometry can detect COPD years before significant dyspnea or other laboratory abnormality occurs. (From Enright PL, Hyatt RE, eds. *Office Spirometry: A Practical Guide to the Selection and Use of Spirometers.* Philadelphia, PA: Lea & Febiger, 1987. Used with permission of Mayo Foundation for Medical Education and Research.)

early testing is shown in Figure 13-1. This shows the typical pattern of development of COPD. Spirometry is the first test to have abnormal results. The innocuous cigarette cough may indicate significant airway obstruction. When confronted with an abnormal test result and appropriate smoking cessation aid, a patient can often be convinced to make a serious attempt to stop smoking, which is a most important step toward improving health. Figure 13-2 shows the average rates of decline in function in smokers with COPD and nonsmokers. The earlier the rapid loss

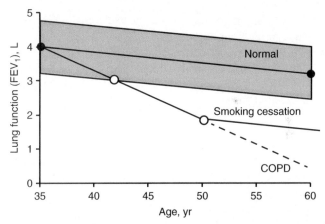

FIG. 13-2 **Normal decline in forced expiratory volume in 1 second (FEV₁) with age contrasted with the accelerated decline in continuing smokers with chronic obstructive pulmonary disease (COPD).** Smoking cessation can halt this rapid decline. (From Enright PL, Hyatt RE, eds. *Office Spirometry: A Practical Guide to the Selection and Use of Spirometers.* Philadelphia, PA: Lea & Febiger, 1987. Used with permission of Mayo Foundation for Medical Education and Research.)

of function can be interrupted in the smoker, the greater will be the life expectancy.

Test: Spirometry before and after bronchodilator.

13B • Chronic Obstructive Pulmonary Disease

Even if the clinical diagnosis of COPD is clear-cut, it is important to quantify the degree of impairment of pulmonary function. An FEV_1 of 50% of predicted portends future disabling disease. An FEV_1 of less than 800 mL predicts future respiratory failure with hypoxia and carbon dioxide retention (hypercapnia).

Repeating spirometry every 1 to 2 years establishes the rate of decline of values such as the FEV_1. The FEV_1 declines an average of 60 mL/y in persons with COPD who continue to smoke,[2] although the range is highly variable,[3] compared with 30 mL/y in normal patients and persons with COPD who quit smoking.[2]

Tests:

1. Initially, spirometry before and after bronchodilator is commonly performed. Although the Global Initiative for Chronic Obstructive Lung Disease (GOLD) guidelines recommend routine use of postbronchodilator values for diagnosis, an argument can be made against routine bronchodilator use in such testing.

2. Measurement of lung volumes (e.g., total lung capacity [TLC], residual volume [RV]) and the diffusing capacity of carbon monoxide (D_{LCO}) are warranted for those with moderate or severe obstruction or symptoms disproportionate to the degree of obstruction.

3. Arterial blood gas studies may be warranted when the FEV_1 is less than 50% predicted.

4. Follow-up testing with spirometry alone or with bronchodilator administration is usually adequate for most patients. Additional measures of lung volumes, DLCO, or other testing can be on an as-needed basis.

13C • Asthma

It is important to be sure that the patient with apparent asthma really has this disease. Remember that "not all that wheezes is asthma." Major airway lesions can cause stridor or wheezing, which may be mistaken for asthma. The flow–volume loop often identifies such lesions (see Section 2K, page 16).

Testing is also important in patients with asthma in remission or with minimal symptoms. This provides a baseline against which to compare results of function tests during an attack and thus quantify the severity of the episode.

Asthmatic patients should be taught to use a peak flow meter. This involves establishing a baseline of peak expiratory flows when asthma is in remission by measuring flows each morning and evening before taking any treatment. They should measure and record peak flows daily.

> **PEARL** ● It is crucial that the patients be taught to use a peak flow meter correctly. They must take a *maximal* inhalation, place their lips around the mouthpiece (a nose clip is not needed), and give a *short, hard blast.* There is no need to make a full exhalation; the exhalation should mimic the quick exhalation used to blow out candles on a birthday cake. They should keep their mouth open during the maneuver. Using the tongue to accelerate flow, as with a blowgun, can falsely increase measures of peak flow.

Having the patient with asthma monitor his or her pulmonary status is extremely important. An exacerbation may be preceded by a decline in peak flow, which the patient may not perceive. By the time the patient becomes symptomatic and dyspneic, flows may have greatly deteriorated. A decrease of about 20% from the symptom-free, baseline peak flow usually means treatments should be reinstated or increased and the physician contacted. It should be impressed on the patient and family that asthma is a serious, *potentially fatal* disease, and that it must be respected and appropriately monitored and treated. Marked airway hyperresponsiveness and highly variable function are harbingers of severe attacks.

Tests:

1. Initial evaluation includes spirometry before and after bronchodilator—determinations of D_{LCO} or lung volumes are optional. If pulmonary function is normal or nearly so and there is any question about the diagnosis, a methacholine challenge or measurement of exhaled nitric oxide (eNO) should be considered (see Chapter 5).
2. For daily monitoring, a peak flow meter is used.
3. Periodic (annual, semiannual, or more frequent) monitoring with spirometry with bronchodilator administration (more often in severe or unstable cases).

13D • Allergic Rhinitis

Allergic rhinitis is often associated with asymptomatic hyperreactive airways. It may evolve into asthma. Thus, establishing a patient's baseline function and airway reactivity may be beneficial.

Tests: Spirometry before and after bronchodilator. If the bronchodilator response is normal but concerns still exist, a methacholine challenge or exhaled nitric oxide (eNO) may be informative (see Chapter 5).

13E • Diffuse Interstitial or Alveolar Pattern on Chest Radiograph

Several disorders can present with these patterns (see Table 12-2, page 101). Pulmonary function tests are performed to answer the following questions: Are the lung volumes decreased and, if so, by how much? Is the diffusing capacity reduced? Is arterial oxygen saturation reduced at rest or with exercise? Not infrequently, oxygen saturation is normal at rest but decreases during exercise. The tests are also used to follow the course of the disease and the response to therapy.

Tests:

1. Spirometry and determination of D_{LCO}, and pulse oximetry at rest and during exercise. Performing spirometry before and after bronchodilator may be useful for initial testing but is probably not needed subsequently if there is no response.
2. Static lung volumes (such as TLC and RV) should be measured at least on first evaluation. Remember that of patients with reduced FVC and normal FEV_1/FVC ratio, only half have a reduced TLC.
3. Measures of lung compliance and recoil pressure at TLC may be available from some advanced laboratories.
4. For routine follow-up visits, spirometry without bronchodilator, and with or without DLCO or oximetry is usually sufficient.

13F • Exertional Dyspnea

In most cases of exertional dyspnea, pulmonary function tests should be performed, even if the major abnormality appears to be nonpulmonary. We have seen patients with dyspnea who have received extensive cardiovascular evaluations before pulmonary function studies were done, and the lungs proved to be the cause of the dyspnea. In addition, exercise-induced bronchospasm, often associated with inhalation of cold air, can be a cause of exertional dyspnea.

Tests: Spirometry before and after bronchodilator and D_{LCO} testing. Determination of oxygen saturation at rest and exercise may be appropriate. For evaluation of exercise-related symptoms, a methacholine challenge may be informative. In difficult cases, cardiopulmonary exercise testing is often helpful (see Section 11F, page 95).

Note: Many patients present with dyspnea, cough, or other respiratory symptoms and are tested before a diagnosis is made. For such patients, an unexplained abnormality, such as a reduction in maximal voluntary ventilation relative to FEV_1 or a peculiar appearing expiratory flow–volume curve, may result in measurement of inspiratory flows or maximal respiratory pressures, thus leading to a correct diagnosis, such as a central airway obstructing process or a neuromuscular disorder.

13G • Chest Tightness

Is the tightness caused by angina or episodic bronchospasm? The distinction is not always easy. Dyspnea is often associated with either disorder. If there is doubt, lung function testing, in addition to cardiac evaluation, is warranted.

Tests: Spirometry before and after bronchodilator. Methacholine challenge or eNO if bronchospasm remains a possibility.

13H • Unexplained Chronic Cough

Some patients have cough that is not related to chronic bronchitis, bronchiectasis, or a current viral infection. The cough may be productive or nonproductive. The most frequent causes are listed in Table 13-1. Obviously, many causes are nonpulmonary. Those in which pulmonary function testing can be helpful are asthma, congestive heart failure, diffuse interstitial disease, and tracheal tumors.

Tests: Spirometry before and after bronchodilator. Expiratory flow–volume curve should be carefully inspected. Inspiratory flow–volume loop should be considered if not performed routinely. Methacholine challenge and DLCO should be considered depending on clinical suspicion.

PEARL ● In patients whose cough follows a pattern of postviral airway hyperresponsiveness syndrome, inhaled or systemic corticosteroids may provide relief, presumably by decreasing eosinophilic airway inflammation that is stimulating cough receptors.

TABLE 13-1 Frequent Causes of Chronic Cough
Postnasal drip
Asthma
Gastroesophageal reflux
Congestive heart failure
Diffuse interstitial disease
Postviral airway hyperresponsiveness
Angiotensin-converting enzyme inhibitor use
Bronchogenic carcinoma
Tracheal tumors
Muscular dystrophy
Ulcerative colitis, Crohn disease
Foreign body

13I • Coronary Artery Disease

Because many patients with coronary artery disease have been smokers, they have an increased risk of also having COPD. And, as noted in Section 12H (page 102), congestive heart failure itself can impair lung function.

Test: Spirometry before and after bronchodilator for cardiac patients with exertional dyspnea.

> **PEARL** • In addition to patients with coronary artery disease, those with hypertension may need to be tested, especially if therapy with non-selective β-adrenergic antagonists is planned. Nonselective β-adrenergic antagonists are usually contraindicated in COPD and asthma, but select-ive β_1-antagonists are generally well tolerated by patients with COPD and most patients with asthma. There is considerable evidence that select-ive β_1-antagonists are underutilized in patients with COPD and coronary disease because of inappropriate fear of adverse consequences from their use. For patients with COPD and asthma, selective β_1-antagonists should be prescribed when they are indicated.

13J • Recurrent Bronchitis or Pneumonia

Not infrequently, asthma and COPD exacerbations are mistaken for recur-rent attacks of bronchitis or pneumonia. This mistake can be avoided by appropriate pulmonary function testing followed by appropriate diagnosis.

Tests: Spirometry before and after bronchodilator. Methacholine chal-lenge may be performed if undetected bronchospasm remains a possibility.

13K • Neuromuscular Disease

There are two reasons for performing pulmonary function tests, including maximal respiratory pressure tests, in patients with neuromuscular dis-ease. First, dyspnea frequently develops in such patients, and it is import-ant to establish the pathogenesis of the complaint. It might be pulmonary or cardiac in origin. Pulmonary function tests help to answer the question. Second, the tests can be useful for following the course of the disease.

Tests: Spirometry before and after bronchodilator, and determination of maximal respiratory pressures. For follow-up visits, maximal respira-tory pressures and slow vital capacity alone.

13L • Occupational and Environmental Exposures

Table 13-2 lists substances and occupations that can produce pulmonary abnormalities reflected in abnormal results of pulmonary tests. Some in-dustries monitor workers' pulmonary function on a regular basis. This testing protects both the worker and the employer.

Tests: Spirometry without bronchodilator. Further testing only if an abnormality is identified.

TABLE 13-2 Occupational and Environmental Exposures That Can Lead to Pulmonary Conditions

Particulates—can precipitate acute coronary events and exacerbations of asthma and chronic obstructive pulmonary disease

Ozone—causes or exacerbates asthma

Nitrogen dioxide—acute lung injury (silo-filler's disease)

Coal dust (coal workers' pneumoconiosis)

Asbestos (pleural plaques, pleural effusion, asbestosis, lung cancer, and mesothelioma)

Silica, quartz (silicosis)

Cotton dust (byssinosis)

Beryllium (chronic beryllium disease, formerly berylliosis)

Talc (talcosis)

Occupational asthma

  Plastics

  Isocyanates

  Animal dander, urine, feces

  Enzyme dusts

  Tea and coffee dust

  Diacetyl (also known as butanedione or butane-2,3-dione) causes "popcorn lung"

  Grain dust

  Wood dusts, especially Western red cedar

Hypersensitivity pneumonitis

  Farmer's lung (exposure to moldy hay)

  Bird-fancier's disease (primarily pigeons, parrots, commercial poultry farms)

  "Hot tub lung"

  Mushroom workers, other moldy dusts

  Humidifier exposure

13M • Systemic Diseases

Several nonpulmonary conditions are frequently associated with altered pulmonary function. Some of the most common ones are listed below, followed by the commonly abnormal pulmonary function test result(s).

1. Rheumatoid arthritis: DLCO reduction is often the first change. Vital capacity may also be reduced, and airflow obstruction occurs in a few cases.

2. Scleroderma (systemic sclerosis): Reduced DLCO is the first change, caused by obliterative vasculopathy not visible by radiography. In some patients, fibrosis can result in reduced lung volumes.

3. Systemic lupus erythematosus: Early decrease in Dlco. Later, volumes may decrease dramatically, producing a "vanishing lung," which may be more related to respiratory muscle weakness than to pulmonary fibrosis.

4. Granulomatosis with polyangiitis (formerly Wegener granulomatosis): Most commonly, central airway lesions are seen on flow–volume curves and spirometry as well as restrictive and obstructive patterns.

5. Polymyositis and dermatomyositis: Patients develop muscle weakness (reduced maximal respiratory pressures) and interstitial disease with low Dlco (most often nonspecific interstitial pneumonia).

6. Cirrhosis of the liver: In some cases, arterial oxygen desaturation is found. This is caused by the development of arteriovenous shunts in the lungs or mediastinum. In many cases, the saturation is lower when the patient is standing (rather than lying), so-called orthodeoxia.

7. Relapsing polychondritis and tracheopathia osteoplastica: Inflammatory degeneration of tracheal and bronchial cartilage can lead to a reduction in inspiratory and expiratory flows, producing an obstructive pattern with characteristic changes in the inspiratory or expiratory flow–volume curve.

8. Sjögren syndrome: As many as half of affected patients have airway obstruction resistant to bronchodilators.

REFERENCES

1. Lin K, Watkins B, Johnson T, et al. Screening for chronic obstructive pulmonary disease using spirometry: summary of the evidence for the U.S. Preventive Services Task Force. *Ann Intern Med* 148:535–543, 2008.
2. Scanlon PD, Connett JE, Waller LA, et al; Lung Health Study Research Group. Smoking cessation and lung function in mild-to-moderate chronic obstructive pulmonary disease. The Lung Health Study. *Am J Respir Crit Care Med* 161:381–390, 2000.
3. Vestbo J, Edwards LD, Scanlon PD, et al; for the ECLIPSE Investigators. Changes in forced expiratory volume in 1 second over time in COPD. *N Engl J Med* 365:1184–1192, 2011.

chapter 14

Interpreting Pulmonary Function Tests

14A • Introduction

This chapter describes our approach to the interpretation of pulmonary function tests. Different experts follow different approaches to the interpretation of pulmonary function tests. There is no universally accepted standard for interpretation. Two older, but commonly cited standards for interpretation are the 1986 American Thoracic Society (ATS) Disability Standard[1] and the 1991 statement of the ATS.[2] In 2005, the ATS and the European Respiratory Society (ERS) updated the pulmonary function standards, including interpretation.[3-7] The ATS/ERS 2005 Interpretation Standard should be the universal standard in North America and Europe, but it has generated unresolved controversies, leaving a variety of opinions. The four main points of concern are (1) the recommendation to use the forced expiratory volume in 1 second to vital capacity (FEV_1/VC) ratio rather than FEV_1/forced expiratory vital capacity (FVC); (2) the *nonspecific pattern* (NSP) with normal FEV_1/FVC ratio, low FVC, and normal total lung capacity (TLC); (3) the isolated reduction in the diffusing capacity of carbon monoxide (D_{LCO}) with normal spirometry and lung volumes; and (4) selection of cut points to define the degree of severity of abnormalities. We will include descriptions of our approach to the points of controversy (see below and Fig. 14-1).

The recommendation for the use of the FEV_1/VC ratio rather than the FEV_1/FVC ratio for the diagnosis of obstruction is based on European[3-7] reference equations. The VC reported is the largest of any VC maneuver regardless of how it was obtained. Hence, the VC is always greater than or equal to the FVC, and, therefore, the FEV_1/VC is always less than or equal to the FEV_1/FVC. If the reference equation used is from a US population and calculates an expected value for FEV_1/FVC, not FEV_1/VC, arbitrarily substituting FEV_1/VC for FEV_1/FVC will cause a systematic bias toward overdiagnosis of obstruction.[4-8]

In the 2005 ATS/ERS flow diagram, the NSP (normal FEV_1/FVC ratio, low FVC, and normal TLC) is interpreted as obstruction (e.g., asthma or chronic bronchitis). In 2009, we published our analysis of this pattern, naming it for the first time (the "nonspecific pattern") and describing its characteristics and clinical associations. At Mayo Clinic, this common pattern accounts for nearly 10% of all pulmonary function tests. As noted in Chapter 3, Section 3G, despite the normal FEV_1/FVC ratio, many cases are, in fact, associated with obstruction, including cases of asthma, other

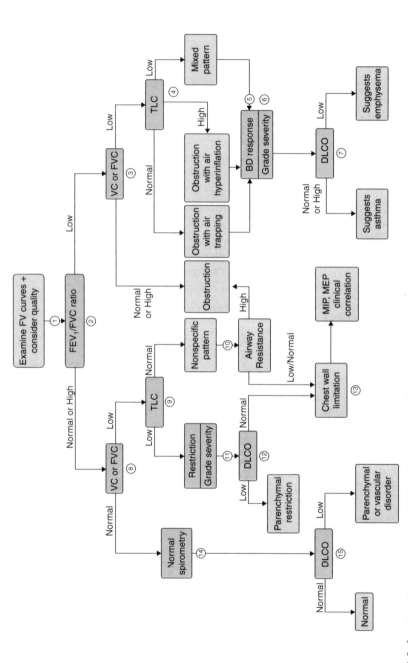

FIG. 14-1 Algorithm for interpretation of results of pulmonary function tests. Numbered steps correspond with numbered steps in text of this chapter. CB, chronic bronchitis; CW, chest wall; D$_{LCO}$, diffusing capacity of carbon monoxide; FEV$_1$, forced expiratory volume in 1 second; ILD, interstitial lung disease; LLN, lower limit of normal; NM, neuromuscular; PV, pulmonary vascular; TLC, total lung capacity; VC, vital capacity. (From *Goldman L, Schafer AI. Goldman-Cecil Medicine.* 25th ed. Philadelphia, PA: Elsevier Saunders; 2015, Figure 85-3.)

forms of airway hyperreactivity, obesity, and chronic obstructive lung disease. We found that a large minority of the cases studied had no evidence of airway obstruction, but rather chest wall limitation (including obesity), muscle weakness, heart failure, cancer, or poor performance.

The isolated reduction in DLCO with normal spirometry and lung volumes is said to be caused by pulmonary vascular (PV) disorders. It is true that PV disorders, such as pulmonary hypertension, can cause this pattern; however, they are relatively uncommon. The most common cause of an isolated reduction in DLCO with normal lung mechanics is emphysema, and it is not always mild when examined with computed tomography. In addition, relatively mild cases of interstitial lung disease often present with low DLCO with lung volumes in the low-normal range.[5–9]

The new ATS/ERS interpretation strategy changes the thresholds defining the severity of obstruction or restriction without providing any rationale for doing so. However, we use the classification of severity shown in Table 14-1, adapted from an earlier ATS standard.[1]

Meanwhile, guidelines for chronic obstructive pulmonary disease (COPD) have been established by numerous groups, most notably, the Global Initiative for Chronic Obstructive Lung Disease (GOLD)[10] and the ACP/ACCP/ATS/ERS.[11] These standards have shifted the grading of severity compared with older standards. This change is said to be motivated by a desire to improve early recognition of disease, but it may prompt prescription of expensive medications, with associated adverse effects for asymptomatic patients, who may not benefit as clearly as more severely affected patients. These concerns are discussed by Enright[12] and Pellegrino et al.[13]

14B • Interpretation 101

General Comments: Be succinct. Your medical colleagues are busy, often so busy they may not carefully read a lengthy interpretation. They may miss a subtle point in a lengthy commentary. So always dictate the most important abnormalities first. Follow with other lesser abnormalities.

Table 14-1 **Impairment and Severity Stratifications**[1]	
Obstruction (60/40/30)[a]	**Restriction (60/50/35)**[b]
FEV$_1$/FVC < LLN and:	FEV$_1$/FVC ≥ LLN and TLC < LLN and:
FEV$_1$ ≥ LLN borderline	FVC < LLN to 60% mild
<LLN to 60% mild	59%–50% moderate
59%–40% moderate	49%–35% severe
39%–30% severe	<35% very severe
<30% very severe	

[a]Numbers in parentheses are forced expiratory volume in 1 second percent predicted.
[b]Numbers in parentheses are forced expiratory vital capacity percent predicted.
FEV$_1$, forced expiratory volume in 1 second; FVC, forced expiratory vital capacity; LLN, lower limit of normal.

Break down abnormalities to brief descriptions (less is more). At the end, combine all remaining normal findings. For example:

"Abnormal. D_{LCO} is severely reduced, consistent with emphysema or other PV or parenchymal process. Spirometry shows only mild obstruction with improved flows after bronchodilator. Lung volumes, inspiratory flows, and resting and exercise oximetry are normal."

The new 2017 ATS Recommendations for a Standardized Pulmonary Function Report advises against reporting or using spirometry data other than FEV_1, FVC, and their ratio, in absolute values and percent predicted, as well as absolute and percent response to bronchodilator, plus FEV_1/slow vital capacity (SVC) and forced expiratory time (FET). Other parameters, such as FEV_3, FEV_6, FEF_{25-75}, and fractional flows, have not been convincingly shown to be useful and are confusing to nonspecialists.[14]

The interpretation Figure 14-1 is from *Goldman-Cecil Medicine*, 25th Edition, 2015. It is adapted from Figure 2 in the 2005 ATS/ERS Interpretation Standard. It is modified to clarify approaches to several controversial points, including those described above. It is then further expanded to cover some issues not addressed by ATS/ERS.[15]

Step 1

Examine the *flow–volume curve* and consider the quality of the multiple maneuvers. Review the technicians' comments regarding the patient's apparent effort or performance, and maneuver quality and any special circumstances that may affect interpretation. Has the patient met the quality standard by performing up to eight maneuvers of which at least three are acceptable and the two best values of FVC and FEV_1 match within 150 mL? If not, I usually preface my interpretive comments with:

"The patient was unable to perform acceptable and repeatable maneuvers, so results may underestimate true lung function."

What does the flow–volume (FV) curve suggest in terms of interpretation? Does it appear to be normal (as in Fig. 14-2)? Does the curve suggest obstruction (scooped out as in Fig. 14-3), restriction (tall, narrow shape, like a witch's hat, in Fig. 14-4), or a special case (see below and Fig. 14-5)? Note that there is a wide range of normal in the degree of

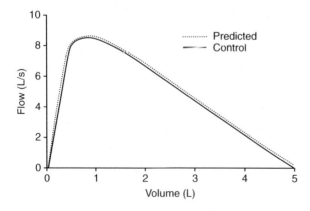

FIG. 14-2 Normal flow–volume curve.

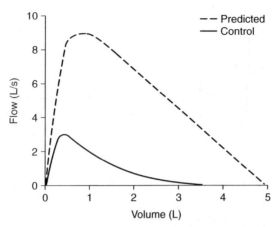

FIG. 14-3 **Flow–volume curve in severe chronic obstructive pulmonary disease.**

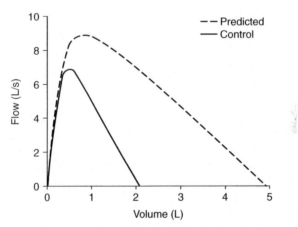

FIG. 14-4 **Flow–volume curve in pulmonary fibrosis.** Note the steep slope and decreased volume.

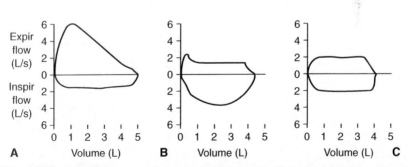

FIG. 14-5 **Typical flow–volume curves associated with lesions of the major airway (carina to mouth).** A. Typical variable extrathoracic lesion. B. Variable intrathoracic lesion. C. Fixed lesion. Expir, expiratory; Inspir, inspiratory.

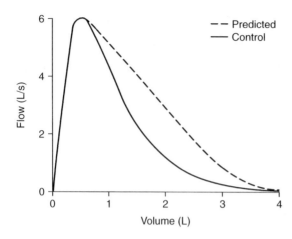

FIG. 14-6 The unusual flow–volume curve in which the forced expiratory volume in 1 second is normal but the forced expiratory flow rate over the middle 50% of the forced expiratory vital capacity is reduced. Note that the peak flow is normal but the lower 70% is very scooped out.

scooping of the flow volume curve. Children and young adults may have a convex curve, whereas older adults (beyond age 50–60) typically have an increasing degree of scooping of the flow volume curve with advancing age (see Fig. 14-6).

Step 2

Is the FEV_1/FVC ratio reduced (below the lower limit normal [LLN]), indicating obstruction (Fig. 14-3)? If so, follow the algorithm to the right (obstruction side). If not, follow the algorithm to the left (restriction side). A normal ratio excludes most obstructive patterns, but an exception is the case of the NSP, in which the FVC and FEV_1 are reduced and the FEV_1/FVC ratio and TLC are normal (see Section 3E, page 30). This is a common pattern affecting 9% to 10% of patients in our laboratory who undergo complete pulmonary function tests (i.e., spirometry, lung volumes, and D_{LCO}). Of patients with the NSP, over half have evidence of obstruction such as responsiveness to bronchodilator (as in Fig. 14-7), increased airway resistance, or clinical evidence of obstructive diseases.

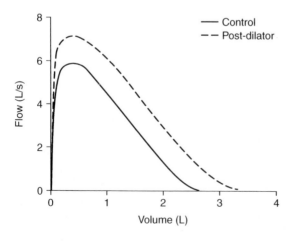

FIG. 14-7 Control curve shows mild reduction in forced expiratory vital capacity (FVC) and forced expiratory volume in 1 second (FEV_1) and a normal FEV_1/FVC ratio. After administration of a bronchodilator, the flow–volume curve (dashed line) shows a parallel shift to the right with an increase in FVC and FEV_1 but no change in the FEV_1/FVC ratio. The patient has occult asthma.

Step 3

Evaluate the FVC. If normal (i.e., >LLN), this is a case of simple obstruction. If <LLN, it may be reduced because of superimposed restriction, that is, a mixed obstructive/restrictive disorder, or, more commonly, it may be reduced because of an increased residual volume, indicating either air trapping or chest wall limitation. If there is no measure of TLC, the distinction between air trapping and a mixed disorder cannot be made (although it may be inferred from radiographic images).

Step 4

Examine the TLC.

a. If the plethysmographic TLC is reduced, one may reliably determine that a mixed obstructive/restrictive disorder is present. In a mixed disorder, you can grade the overall severity of impairment from the FEV_1 percent predicted. You can grade the severity of the restrictive component from the TLC percent predicted. The severity of the obstructive component can be determined by dividing the FEV_1 percent predicted by the TLC percent predicted (expressed as a fraction).[16] See Case 30 in the illustrative cases, Chapter 15.

b. If a gas-dilution TLC (He dilution or N_2 washout) is reduced, it may indicate a restrictive process, or may be reduced because lung volumes are underestimated because of poorly communicating airspaces, particularly in patients with extensive emphysema.

c. If TLC is normal, this is a case of simple obstruction, the severity of which can be judged from the FEV_1 percent predicted.

d. If TLC is increased, some interpreters will identify hyperinflation. The definition of hyperinflation and the degree of increase required to identify it are not addressed by the ATS/ERS standards. I use a cut point of 125% to 130% predicted to identify hyperinflation. In addition, if plethysmographic TLC is greater than 150% predicted, I question the validity of the measurement and asked the technicians to reanalyze the panting loops. TLC may be overestimated if the panting frequency is too fast or if the angles of the loops are measured incorrectly.

e. If TLC is not increased but residual volume (RV) is greater than the upper limit normal (ULN) and the RV/TLC ratio is greater than ULN, some interpreters will identify air trapping. This is also not discussed by the ATS/ERS standards. Remember that although air trapping is often caused by airway closure at low lung volumes, it may also be caused by muscle weakness or chest wall limitation near RV, unrelated to airway disorders.

f. If lung volumes were not measured—do not fail to comment on a low FVC in spirometry. It may be important and is easy to overlook. I usually say:
"Abnormal. Mild/moderate/severe obstruction with reduced vital capacity. The low vital capacity may be due to air trapping, but

a superimposed restrictive process cannot be ruled out without measurement of lung volumes."

Sometimes, a previous test will clarify the cause of the reduced VC, in which case:

"Abnormal. Mild/moderate/severe obstruction with reduced vital capacity (the latter has previously been shown to be due to air trapping, not superimposed restriction)."

Step 5

Examine the Response to Bronchodilator. A positive response to bronchodilator is defined by ATS/ERS as an increase in either FEV_1 or FVC by 12% and 200 mL. I usually comment if a positive response is unusually large. A large bronchodilator response is predictive of more exacerbations and more rapid decline in lung function. Experts disagree on fine points, such as what to call lesser degrees of response. Note that a positive bronchodilator response does not always yield an improvement in FEV_1/FVC ratio. In fact the ratio may be the same or lower after a positive bronchodilator response (see Fig. 14-7). Be careful to address whether a volume response (increase in FVC but not FEV_1) is caused by prolonged expiratory effort alone (as indicted by a longer FET).

Step 6

Grade Severity of Obstruction. Prior to 2005, most pulmonary function interpreters graded severity of obstruction on the basis of prebronchodilator FEV_1 percent predicted. There was a wide consensus not to grade on the basis of the FEV_1/FVC ratio. Since 2005, ATS/ERS recommends grading severity of obstruction on the basis of postbronchodilator FEV_1 percent predicted. GOLD Guidelines recommend the same for patients with COPD. Dr. Hyatt said that is like grading the severity of hypertension on the basis of blood pressure while on therapy, and I agree.

    Obstruction algorithm: If FEV_1/FVC ratio < LLN, the degree of obstruction is based on the FEV_1 percent predicted, either pre- or postbronchodilator.

TABLE 14-2 **Two Algorithms for Grading the Severity of Obstruction**	
For all, FEV1/FVC < LLN	
Adapted from 1986 ATS Disability Standard	ATS/ERS 2005 Interpretation Standard
FEV_1/FVC < LLN and FEV_1 ≥ LLN borderline	
FEV_1 60% to < LLN mild	FEV_1/FVC < LLN and FEV_1 > 70% mild
FEV_1 40% to 59% moderate	FEV_1 60% to 69% moderate
	FEV_1 50% to 59% moderately severe
FEV_1 30% to 39% severe	FEV_1 35% to 49% severe
FEV_1 <30% very severe	FEV_1 <35% very severe

It is possible to grade the severity of COPD on the basis of GOLD stages, but that requires more clinical information than we are provided with for most patients in the pulmonary function laboratory.

Optional Step

Examine the maximal voluntary ventilation if you have one.

1. The maximal voluntary ventilation (MVV) is not commonly measured by most laboratories, but we measure it routinely. It will change in most cases in a manner similar to the FEV_1. With a *normal* FEV_1, a normal MVV should be expected ($FEV_1 \times 40$ = predicted MVV). Consider the lower limit for MVV to be $FEV_1 \times 30$, that is, in both obstructive and restrictive disorders, the MVV is usually greater than $FEV_1 \times 30$.

2. If the FEV_1 is *normal* but the MVV is *reduced* below the lower limit, consider the following possibilities:

   a. Neuromuscular weakness—The MVV is reasonably sensitive to weakness, although neither as sensitive nor as specific as maximal respiratory pressures, which can be added as the next appropriate tests (see Chapter 9).

   b. Major airway lesion—MVV is reduced relative to FEV_1 if inspiratory flow is reduced (Figure 14-5A and C); to evaluate this, the flow–volume loop, including inspiratory flows, needs to be evaluated. The next step may include imaging or direct visualization of the airway by bronchoscopy or laryngoscopy.

   c. Poor patient performance—due to lack of coordination, fatigue, coughing, or unwillingness to give maximal effort (best judged by the technician, so technician's comments should always be considered).

Step 7

Examine the D_{LCO}.

1. Is the D_{LCO} *reduced*? D_{LCO} is commonly reduced in patients with a gas exchange abnormality (e.g., emphysema, idiopathic pulmonary fibrosis, and other parenchymal or vascular processes or heart failure). In current and former smokers with obstruction, a low D_{LCO} is most often caused by emphysema, whereas in asthma and some cases of chronic obstructive bronchitis, D_{LCO} is usually normal. It is worthwhile to point out the likelihood of emphysema, particularly for patients who are current smokers and may benefit from motivation to quit. A typical interpretation might say: "Abnormal. Severe obstruction with hyperinflation. Flows improve after bronchodilator, suggesting an element of reversible obstruction. D_{LCO} is severely reduced, consistent with emphysema or other pulmonary vascular or parenchymal process. Anemia may contribute to the low D_{LCO}." If the patient is a never smoker, the possibility of emphysema can be dropped from

the interpretation. The cut points for severity of reduction in DLCO have never varied among standards! Mild is below the LLN, moderate is < 60%, and severe < 40%. DLCO should be adjusted for low hemoglobin for anemic patients (showing both the unadjusted DLCO and the hemoglobin value used for adjustment).

2. Is the DLCO *normal*? In obstructive disorders, this suggests predominantly airway disease, such as asthma or chronic bronchitis, with relatively normal lung parenchyma. Is the DLCO *increased*? This occurs mainly in patients with asthma and in obese patients. Other conditions are less common, including alveolar hemorrhage, polycythemia or left-to-right intracardiac shunt, heart failure, nonresting state, and supine position.[17]

Step 8

Restriction Side of Algorithm—Evaluate FVC or VC. If the FEV_1/FVC ratio is normal or high and the FV curve does not indicate otherwise, consider the possibility of a restrictive disorder. Consider the FVC and other measures of VC. If it is (or they are) reduced, this may indicate restriction. This has been called PRISm (preserved ratio impaired spirometry) by the COPDGene Investigators[18] and accounts for about 20% of patients in our laboratory. The appropriate next step is to examine TLC. If only spirometry is available, further evaluation depends on either obtaining measurement of TLC or imaging or clinical assessment. If no current or prior TLC is available, it can only be said that spirometry is consistent with a restrictive or a nonspecific abnormality. It should be noted that in our laboratory, of patients with "spirometric restriction" or PRISm, about 50% have a low TLC. The other half have a normal TLC and, hence, the NSP.

Step 9

Evaluate TLC.

a. If TLC is abnormally low, this is a restrictive disorder (see Step 11). Pulmonary function experts have argued for years over whether to grade the severity of impairment on the basis of reduction in TLC or FVC and what cut points to use. The 2005 ATS/ERS Interpretation Standard recommended FEV_1 without explanation or rationale. They recommend cut points of LLN, 70%, 60%, 50%, 35% for mild, moderate, moderately severe, severe, and very severe. In our laboratory, we still use cut points for FVC or TLC on the basis of 1986 ATS Disability Standard, with LLN%, 60%, 50%, 35% for mild, moderate, severe, and very severe, respectively.

b. If FVC is reduced but TLC is normal, this is not restriction (see Step 10). We have called this the NSP.[19,20] Although very common, this pattern was unnamed until 2009. In the 2005 ATS/ERS Interpretation Algorithm, it was called obstruction with little

TABLE 14-3 **Two Algorithms for Grading the Severity of Restriction**	
For all, FEV$_1$/FVC > LLN	
From 1986 ATS Disability Standard	ATS/ERS 2005 Interpretation Standard
TLC or FVC 60% to LLN mild	FEV$_1$ < LLN to 70% mild
TLC or FVC 50% to 59% moderate	FEV$_1$ 60% to 69% moderate
	FEV$_1$ 50% to 59% moderately severe
TLC or FVC 35% to 49% severe	FEV$_1$ 35% to 49% severe
TLC or FVC < 35% very severe	FEV$_1$ <35% very severe
	FEV$_1$ <35% very severe

explanation. In the descriptions of NSP, it is noted that it is commonly (>50%) associated with evidence of obstruction, despite the normal FEV$_1$/FVC ratio. But in a sizable subset (30%–50%), there is evidence of chest wall limitation (particularly obesity), muscle weakness, cancer, heart failure, or poor performance. The pattern is fairly stable over 3 to 5 years of follow-up.[20] When we identify the NSP, we routinely measure airway resistance (Step 10). If elevated (about half the time), it suggests an obstructive disorder. If normal, it suggests chest wall limitation, muscle weakness, or poor performance (Step 13).

   c. If the TLC percent predicted is reduced (Step 11), and the FVC percent predicted is reduced to a greater degree, this may be a complex restrictive case, which is defined by a TLC < LLN and a difference between TLC percent predicted and FVC percent predicted ≥10%. For example, a patient may have a TLC of 68% predicted and an FVC of 38% predicted. Depending on the interpreter, that might be called mild restriction or severe restriction, or even mild-to-severe restriction! This dilemma led to the study of the complex restrictive disorder (see Section 3H). These cases make up about one-third of all restrictive cases, or 4% of all complete pulmonary function tests. The "something else" contributing to the abnormality may be muscle weakness, chest wall limitation (including obesity), poor performance, or occult obstruction (see also Table 12-1; Section 9D).[21] In many cases, chest imaging, measurements of maximal respiratory pressures, or additional clinical assessments are helpful.

Step 12

Examine Dlco. If D$_{LCO}$ is abnormal in a patient with restriction, it supports the likelihood of a parenchymal restrictive process such as idiopathic pulmonary fibrosis or asbestosis. In such cases, the D$_{LCO}$ is usually reduced to a degree similar to the degree of restriction or sometimes worse. On the other hand, if the DLCO is relatively preserved, or even normal, it suggests that the restriction may be caused by chest wall limitation (Step 13) rather than a pulmonary parenchymal abnormality. If so, measurement of maximal respiratory pressures can distinguish muscle weakness from other causes of chest wall limitation. Clinical history and imaging are often enlightening. Lung resection with otherwise healthy lungs usually results in relative sparing of DLCO.

Step 14

Normal Spirometry. If FEV_1/FVC ratio, FVC, and FEV_1 are all normal, spirometry is normal (generally ignore FEF_{25-75}, which may be low, particularly in elderly patients). Some consideration can be made for abnormal FV curves (see Fig. 14-5). If TLC is reduced, consider a mild restrictive disorder.

Step 15

Examine Dlco. If spirometry and lung volumes are normal but DLCO is reduced, you have an isolated reduction in DLCO. This is said to imply PV disorders by the 2005 ATS/ERS Interpretation Standard. In fact, it is more often caused by emphysema or interstitial disease or a combination of both (combined pulmonary fibrosis and emphysema—CPFE).[22] PV disorders such as scleroderma, primary or secondary pulmonary hypertension, recurrent emboli, and vasculitides are less common as an explanation. It should be noted that although DLCO may be reduced in pulmonary hypertension, it is insensitive for detecting pulmonary hypertension. Chemotherapeutic agents can also produce this finding, and DLCO is often used to monitor for an adverse pulmonary effect of chemotherapy.

Examine *other test results* that you may have available. They should confirm the interpretation at which you have already arrived and fit the patterns in Table 12-1.

Funny Looking FV Curves

The FV curve can appear unusual for a variety of reasons, including several normal variants and several distinct clinical abnormalities. Most people have a very reproducible FV curve, when multiple maximal expiratory efforts are performed. The normal FV curve is roughly triangular, but some people have distinct bumps on their FV curves. Most often these are in the upper one-fourth to one-half of the curve. The bumps usually represent transition points when the point of flow limitation moves from the trachea to the mainstem bronchi or smaller airways. Some patients, usually young adults or adolescents with normal lung function, have a prominent tracheal plateau (see Fig. 2-6H and Cases 1 and 38), which signifies flow limitation in the trachea at lung volumes at which flow is normally more limited in the peripheral airways. Thus, a tracheal plateau is a sign of healthy peripheral airways. Another normal variant is a convex FV curve, which is typical of children, but which can be an indicator of muscle weakness or poor performance in an adult (Fig. 2-6D).

Some maneuver errors can be identified from examination of the FV curve. These include slow start, poor blast, cough, or interruption in the first second and early termination of effort (see examples in Fig. 2-6).

Finally, a variety of abnormalities can be identified by examination of the FV curve, particularly in comparing the inspiratory and expiratory curves. These include the following:

a. A plateau on the FV curve may indicate a central airway obstructive process. Upper airway or extrathoracic (i.e., above the thoracic inlet) lesions affect inspiration more than expiration (see Fig. 14-5A). Intrathoracic (i.e., below the thoracic inlet) lesions affect expiration more than inspiration (see Fig. 14-5B). A fixed central obstructive lesion (such as a tracheal stricture or stenosis) limits inspiratory and expiratory flows equally (Fig. 14-5C).

b. A sawtooth abnormality usually affects the higher flows on the FV curve. This has a higher frequency than coughing. It indicates redundant tissue in the upper airway and is associated with increased risk of obstructive sleep apnea (See Chapter 15, Case 13).[23]

Methacholine Challenge

This is positive if there is a 20% or greater decrease in FEV_1 after a threshold concentration, or dose, of methacholine. In the past, the threshold concentration was 25 mg/mL, but various standards have recommended lower thresholds (as low as 4 or 8 mg/mL) to increase test specificity. Calculation of dose requires knowledge of the output of the nebulizer and some assumptions about tidal breathing patterns and aerosol deposition. The reality of those assumptions is unknown, as is the respirable output of most nebulizers, so our laboratory continues to report results in terms of concentration.

Elements needed for clinical diagnosis of asthma include: (1) evidence of airway hyperresponsiveness, (2) obstruction varying over time, and (3) evidence of airway inflammation. Thus, as always, the results of laboratory testing should be evaluated in the clinical context on the basis of pretest probability of disease, in this case asthma.

Maximal Respiratory Pressures ("Bugles")

These are used to assess respiratory muscle strength. If low, they indicate *muscle weakness* or *poor performance*. Inspiratory pressure is mostly a function of diaphragmatic strength. Tetraplegics show reduced expiratory pressures with inspiratory pressures (diaphragm) relatively preserved. Diaphragmatic paralysis is the opposite (see Chapter 9 for fuller discussion).

Obesity

Obesity usually has only modest effects on pulmonary function. The most consistent abnormality is a reduced expiratory reserve volume (ERV, the difference between functional residual capacity and RV). The increased chest wall impedance can cause a restrictive pattern in some very obese patients. On average, a person with a body mass index of 35 will have a 5% to 10% reduction in FVC compared with someone with a body mass index of 25, so typically would not be interpreted as being outside the normal range. TLC is usually not reduced to the same degree as FVC. Obese people may wheeze when they breathe near RV, sometimes called pseudo-asthma. DLCO is usually normal or increased. Additional effects of obesity on pulmonary function are discussed in Section 12I and Table 12-1.[24]

REFERENCES

1. American Thoracic Society. Evaluation of impairment/disability secondary to respiratory disorders. *Am Rev Respir Dis* 133:1205–1209, 1986.
2. American Thoracic Society. Lung function testing: selection of reference values and interpretative strategies. *Am Rev Respir Dis* 144:1202–1218, 1991.
3. Miller MR, Crapo R, Hankinson J, et al. General considerations for lung function testing. *Eur Respir J* 26:153–161, 2005.
4. Miller MR, Hankinson J, Brusasco V, et al. Standardisation of spirometry. *Eur Respir J* 26:319–338, 2005.
5. Wanger J, Clausen JL, Coates A, et al. Standardisation of the measurement of lung volumes. *Eur Respir J* 26:511–522, 2005.
6. Graham BL, Brusasco V, Burgos F, et al. 2017 ERS/ATS standards for single-breath carbon monoxide uptake in the lung. *Eur Respir J* 49:1600–1616, 2017.
7. Pellegrino R, Viegi G, Brusasco V, et al. Interpretative strategies for lung function tests. *Eur Respir J* 26:948–968, 2005.
8. Hankinson JL, Odencrantz JR, Fedan KB. Spirometric reference values from a sample of the general U.S. population. *Am J Respir Crit Care Med* 159:179–187, 1999.
9. Aduen JF, Zisman DA, Mobin SI, et al. Retrospective study of pulmonary function tests in patients presenting with isolated reduction in single-breath diffusion capacity: implications for the diagnosis of combined obstructive and restrictive lung disease. *Mayo Clin Proc* 82:48–54, 2007.
10. GOLD website. https://goldcopd.org/.
11. http://www.thoracic.org/statements/resources/copd/179full.pdf.
12. Enright P. Flawed interpretative strategies for lung function tests harm patients [editorial]. *Eur Respir J* 27:1322–1323, 2006.
13. Pellegrino R, Brusasco V, Crapo RO, et al. From the authors [editorial]. *Eur Respir J* 27:1323–1324, 2006.
14. Culver BH, Graham BL, Coates AL, et al. Recommendations for a standardized pulmonary function report. *Am J Respir Crit Care Med* 196:1463–1472, 2017.
15. Scanlon PD. Respiratory function: mechanisms and testing. In: Goldman L, Schafer AI, eds. *Goldman-Cecil Medicine*, 25th ed. Philadelphia, PA: Elsevier Saunders, 2015.
16. Gardner ZS, Ruppel GL, Kaminsky DA. Grading the severity of obstruction in mixed obstructive-restrictive lung disease. *Chest* 140(3):598–603, 2011.
17. Saydain G, Beck KC, Decker PA, Cowl CT, Scanlon PD. Clinical significance of elevated diffusing capacity. *Chest* 125(2):446–452, 2004.
18. Wan ES, Castaldi PJ, Cho MH, et al. Epidemiology, genetics, and subtyping of preserved ratio impaired spirometry (PRISm) in COPDGene. *Resp Res* 15:89, 2014.
19. Hyatt RE, Cowl CT, Bjoraker JA, Scanlon PD. Conditions associated with an abnormal nonspecific pattern of pulmonary function tests. *Chest* 135(2):419–424, 2009.
20. Iyer VN, Schroeder DR, Parker KO, Hyatt RE, Scanlon PD. The nonspecific pulmonary function test: longitudinal follow-up and outcomes. *Chest* 139(4):878–886, 2011.
21. Clay RD, Iyer VN, Reddy DR, Siontis B, Scanlon PD. The "complex restrictive" pulmonary function pattern. *Chest* 152:1258–1265, 2017.
22. Cottin V, Nunes H, Brillet PY, et al. Combined pulmonary fibrosis and emphysema: a distinct underrecognised entity. *Eur Respir J* 26:586–593, 2005.
23. Bourne MH, Scanlon PD, Schroeder DR, Olson EJ. The sawtooth sign is predictive of obstructive sleep apnea. *Sleep Breath* 21:469–474, 2017.
24. Jones RL, Nzekwu MM. The effects of body mass index on lung volumes. *Chest* 130:827–833, 2006.

chapter 15

Illustrative Cases

15A • Introduction

The cases presented in this chapter demonstrate many of the points made in the preceding chapters. A few examples are unusual cases, but most present problems that are commonly evaluated in the pulmonary function laboratory.

For most of the cases, the flow–volume curve should be studied first. Consider whether obstruction or restriction or some other abnormality can be identified. After that, the measurements should be reviewed looking first at the ratio of the forced expiratory volume in 1 second to the forced expiratory vital capacity (FEV_1/FVC ratio) to distinguish obstruction from restriction. Then, review the other data to determine whether they support or change the initial impression and to provide further detail. Usually, several questions will be posed, and an attempt should be made to answer them before the answers and discussion are read. In the tables, the normal predicted value, observed value, and the percentage of the predicted value are listed. Abnormal values that are outside the normal range are indicated by an asterisk (*). Interpretations are provided after the case discussion. They follow (mostly) the 2005 American Thoracic Society/European Respiratory Society recommendations except where noted or as discussed in Chapter 14, pages 113–115. The types of cases are listed on pages 227 and 228.

CASE 1

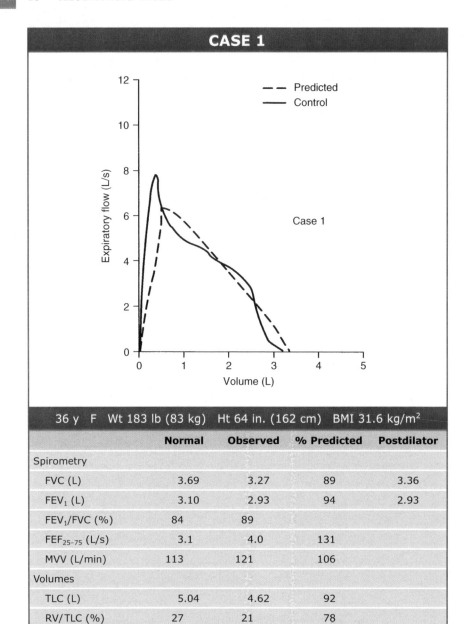

36 y F Wt 183 lb (83 kg) Ht 64 in. (162 cm) BMI 31.6 kg/m²				
	Normal	**Observed**	**% Predicted**	**Postdilator**
Spirometry				
FVC (L)	3.69	3.27	89	3.36
FEV₁ (L)	3.10	2.93	94	2.93
FEV₁/FVC (%)	84	89		
FEF₂₅₋₇₅ (L/s)	3.1	4.0	131	
MVV (L/min)	113	121	106	
Volumes				
TLC (L)	5.04	4.62	92	
RV/TLC (%)	27	21	78	
D_LCO (mL/min/mm Hg)	24	24	100	

Questions

1. Does the patient have ventilatory limitation?

2. Do the test values support your impression?

3. Is the configuration of the flow–volume curve normal?

CASE 1

Answers

1. There is no ventilatory limitation.

2. The test values are all normal.

3. Over most of the vital capacity, flow decreases in a relatively gradual, steady manner. However, at 2.4 L of expired volume, there is a "knee" in the curve after which flow decreases more rapidly. This contour is not caused by a major airway lesion but is a normal variant that occurs mostly in young nonsmokers, especially women. This patient had never smoked. This shape is caused by the transition of the point of flow limitation moving peripherally as lung volumes decrease. The "knee" represents the lung volume at which the point of flow limitation moves to the mainstem bronchi, then moves further toward the periphery as lung volume decreases. This is called a *tracheal plateau*. It can be considered a sign of healthy peripheral airways (see Fig. 2-6H).

   Interpretation: "Normal spirometry, lung volumes, and DLco with no acute bronchodilator response. The shape of the flow–volume curve is a normal variant."

CASE 2

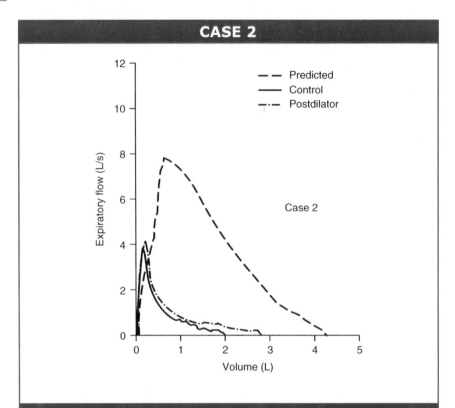

71 y M Wt 195 lb (88 kg) Ht 69 in. (175 cm) BMI 28.7 kg/m²				
	Normal	**Observed**	**% Predicted**	**Postdilator**
Spirometry				
FVC (L)	4.29	1.94*	45	2.76
FEV₁ (L)	3.29	1.03*	31	1.25
FEV₁/FVC (%)	77	53*		
FEF₂₅₋₇₅ (L/s)	2.8	0.4*	15	0.5
MVV (L/min)	125	51*	41	
Volumes				
TLC (L)	6.61	9.37*	142	
RV/TLC (%)	35	75*	214	
DLCO (mL/min/mm Hg)	25	10*	40	

Comments and Questions

This patient had a smoking history of 74 pack-years and was still smoking. He complained of progressive breathlessness and wheezing on mild exertion. His parents both had smoking-related emphysema, and his father died of lung cancer.

1. How would you interpret this test?
2. Can you make a statement as to the patient's underlying lung disease?
3. Does the DLCO suggest anything?

CASE 2

Answers

1. The patient has severe ventilatory limitation on an obstructive basis. Hyperinflation is present with an increased total lung capacity (TLC). The increased residual volume (RV)/TLC ratio indicates air trapping, which is virtually always seen with hyperinflation. Hyperinflation is less common and is not always seen in patients with air trapping. Flows improve, along with a large reduction in air trapping, after bronchodilator.

2. If only spirometry results were available, it would be appropriate to say, "There is severe ventilatory limitation on an obstructive basis, but a small restrictive component cannot be ruled out without a measurement of total lung capacity." Of course, if a chest radiograph showed hyperinflation, then one would be relatively certain that the abnormalities were all obstructive.

3. In this case with the hyperinflation and obstruction, the low D_{LCO} is consistent with emphysema, and computed tomography (CT) would be expected to confirm this. In Case 20 (page 173), in which the TLC is very low and the slope of the flow–volume curve is steep, the low D_{LCO} probably reflects the presence of interstitial disease. Usually, an appropriate comment for a low D_{LCO} is, "the low D_{LCO} suggests a parenchymal or vascular abnormality."

Interpretation: "Abnormal. Very severe obstruction with improved flows after bronchodilator. Lung volumes show hyperinflation. The moderate-to-severe reduction in D_{LCO} is consistent with emphysema or other parenchymal or vascular process or anemia."

CASE 3

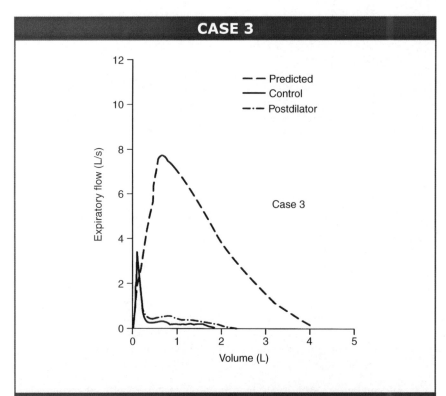

69 y M Wt 143 lb (65 kg) Ht 68 in. (173 cm) BMI 21.7 kg/m²				
	Normal	**Observed**	**% Predicted**	**Postdilator**
Spirometry				
FVC (L)	4.11	1.73*	42	2.30*
FEV$_1$ (L)	3.18	0.48*	15	0.63*
FEV$_1$/FVC (%)	77	28*		
FEF$_{25-75}$ (L/s)	2.8	0.2*	8	0.3*
MVV (L/min)	124	24*	19	
Volumes				
TLC (L)	6.39	7.62	119	
RV/TLC (%)	36	71*	197	
D$_{LCO}$ (mL/min/mm Hg)	25	12*	47	

Questions

1. How would you interpret this test?
2. What would you predict the predilator maximal voluntary ventilation (MVV) would be?

CASE 3

Answers

1. This is a classic case of very severe obstructive disease with very severe obstruction, air trapping, and moderately reduced D_{LCO}. There is a "volume response" to bronchodilator, meaning FEV_1 increases by less than 200 mL, but vital capacity increases, not just because of longer expiratory time. The reduced D_{LCO} suggests an element of anatomic emphysema. The plateau in the flow–volume curve is typical of severe chronic obstructive pulmonary disease and should not be mistaken for a variable intrathoracic airway lesion.

2. The predilator MVV would be predicted to be 40×0.48 $(FEV_1) = 19$ L/min (see Section 2I). The measured value was 24 L/min. This difference does not mean that the FEV_1 was in error but merely points out the limitation of the prediction equation and the variability in the relationship between the MVV and FEV_1. Of interest, during an exercise study done on the same day, the patient achieved a minute ventilation of 36 L/min. Thus, predicting maximal ventilation during exercise from the FEV_1 or MVV may also not be exact.

   Interpretation: "Abnormal. Very severe obstruction with air trapping and moderately reduced D_{LCO}. The increased vital capacity after bronchodilator indicates reduced air trapping."

CASE 4

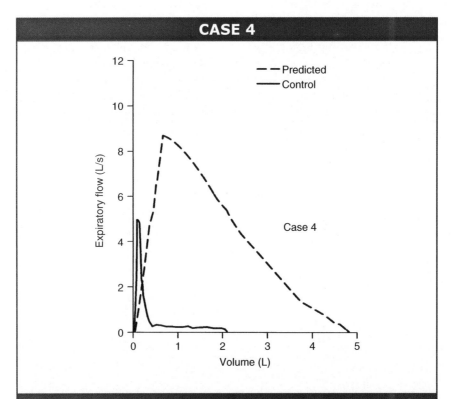

67 y M Wt 189 lb (86 kg) Ht 71 in. (180 cm) BMI 26.5 kg/m²				
	Normal	**Observed**	**% Predicted**	**Postdilator**
Spirometry				
FVC (L)	4.79	2.06*	43	2.67
FEV$_1$ (L)	3.67	0.56*	15	0.75
FEV$_1$/FVC (%)	77	27*		
FEF$_{25-75}$ (L/s)	31	0.2*	6	
MVV (L/min)	136	29*	21	
Volumes				
TLC (L)	7.02	8.64*	123	
RV/TLC (%)	32	69*	216	
D$_{LCO}$ (mL/min/mm Hg)	27	21	79	

Comments and Questions

This 67-year-old man had a 59 pack-year smoking history and was still smoking 10 cigarettes per day. He had complained 5 years previously of shortness of breath while walking on a level surface. His dyspnea, often accompanied by wheezing, had become progressively worse, to the point that he now can walk less than one block before stopping.

1. How would you describe the flow–volume curve?
2. Do the test results support your impression? (Incidentally, the postbronchodilator flow–volume curve is not shown for the sake of clarity, but it did show higher flows and volumes.)

CASE 4

Answers

1. Flows are markedly reduced, and the curve is typical of obstruction. Thus, "severe ventilatory limitation secondary to airway obstruction" would be correct.

2. The increased TLC and RV are consistent with this interpretation, as are the markedly reduced FEV_1 and flows across the range of the vital capacity.

   The D_{LCO} is in the low-normal range, which argues against significant anatomic emphysema. This is a good example of a patient with chronic bronchitis who responds to a bronchodilator and has desaturation with exercise. Not shown was the oximetry result—a resting oxygen saturation of 94% that decreased to 86% with mild exercise.

   Interpretation: "Abnormal. Very severe obstruction with air trapping and borderline bronchodilator response. D_{LCO} is low normal. Resting oximetry is normal, but saturation decreases during exercise."

CASE 5

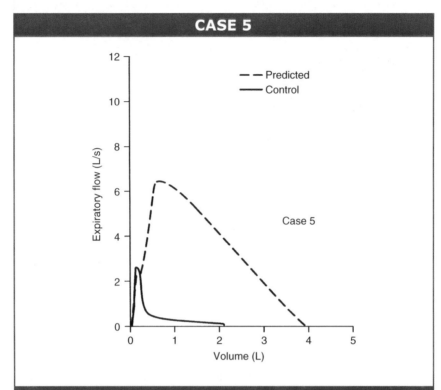

29 y   F   Wt 110 lb (50 kg)   Ht 65 in. (165 cm)   BMI 18.4 kg/m²

	Normal	Observed	% Predicted	Postdilator
Spirometry				
FVC (L)	3.93	2.39*	61	2.86
FEV$_1$ (L)	3.34	0.62*	19	0.67
FEV$_1$/FVC (%)	85	26*		
FEF$_{25-75}$ (L/s)	3.4	0.2*	6	0.2
MVV (L/min)	119	28*	23	
Volumes				
TLC (L)	5.18	6.63	128	
RV/TLC (%)	24	59*	246	
D$_{LCO}$ (mL/min/mm Hg)	25	7*	28	

Comment and Questions

This young woman was a nonsmoker with no history of asthma.

1. How would you grade the limitation based on the flow–volume curve?
2. Do the spirometry results support your impression? (The postdilator curve is not shown because it could not be distinguished from the control curve.)
3. Are the volumes and DLCO also consistent?
4. What is unusual about this case?

CASE 5

Answers

1. The flow–volume curve shows severe ventilatory limitation because of an obstructive process. The shape of the curve is characteristic of obstruction.

2. Spirometry results are consistent with very severe obstruction.

3. The high-normal TLC and reduced D_{LCO} are also consistent with severe obstruction. The low D_{LCO} suggests a parenchymal abnormality, such as emphysema.

4. The patient was a nonsmoker with no history of asthma. This degree of obstruction in such a young person is uncommon. One possibility would be α_1-antitrypsin deficiency, but results of blood tests were normal. On open-lung biopsy, the patient was found to have lymphangioleiomyomatosis. This is a rare disease in which there is proliferation of atypical smooth muscle throughout the peribronchial, perivascular, and perilymphatic regions of the lung. Pulmonary infiltrates were prominent on chest radiography (these do not occur in α_1-antitrypsin deficiency) and contribute to the reduction in the D_{LCO}.

   Interpretation: "Abnormal. Very severe obstruction with air trapping and no response to bronchodilator. D_{LCO} is severely reduced consistent with the pulmonary vascular or parenchymal process."

CASE 6

62 y F Wt 90 lb (40 kg) Ht 63 in. (160 cm) BMI 15.6 kg/m²				
	Normal	**Observed**	**% Predicted**	**Postdilator**
Spirometry				
FVC (L)	2.6	1.95*	75	1.95
FEV$_1$ (L)	1.9	0.35*	18	0.35
FEV$_1$/FVC (%)	74	18*		
FEF$_{25-75}$ (L/s)	2.9	0.3*	10	
MVV (L/min)	62	16*	25	
Volumes				
TLC (L)	4.6	5.5	120	
RV/TLC (%)	43	66*	153	
D$_{LCO}$ (mL/min/mm Hg)	22	8*	36	

Comments and Questions

This 62-year-old woman complained of weight loss, rectal bleeding, nervousness, and some shortness of breath on exertion. She noted dyspnea after recovery from influenza. She had never smoked and had no family history of respiratory disease. The chest radiograph revealed decreased lung markings in both bases. The TLC measured with the nitrogen washout technique was 1 L less than the plethysmographic TLC reported here.

1. How would you describe these data?
2. Are there any additional tests you would order?

CASE 6

Answers

1. The test results are consistent with severe airway obstruction with hyperinflation, yet dyspnea was not a major complaint. The chest radiograph and the low diffusing capacity suggest the presence of emphysema with an unusual basal distribution.

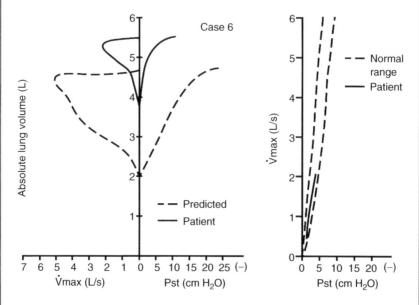

2. Testing for α_1-antitrypsin deficiency revealed very low enzyme levels and that she was homozygous for the Z allele. Special mechanics studies were ordered. Note the severe loss of lung recoil and hyperinflation. The maximal flow static recoil (MFSR) curve lies in the normal range, consistent with pure emphysema. CL_{stat} was increased (0.389 L/cm H_2O), whereas CL_{dyn} was low (0.132 L/cm H_2O) (see Section 7B). Resistance was increased at 6.2 cm $H_2O/L/s$.

Interpretation: "Very severe obstruction with air trapping, no bronchodilator response, and severely reduced DLCO, consistent with a pulmonary parenchymal or vascular process. The MFSR curve is within the normal range, indicating parenchymal loss of recoil as the cause for airflow obstruction."

CASE 7

56 y M Wt 162 lb (73.6 kg) Ht 66 in. (168 cm) BMI 26.1 kg/m²				
	Normal	**Observed**	**% Predicted**	**Postdilator**
Spirometry				
FVC (L)	3.3	4.67	141	4.67
FEV$_1$ (L)	2.4	1.72*	72	2.02
FEV$_1$/FVC (%)	73	37*		
FEF$_{25-75}$ (L/s)	3.4	0.7*	21	
MVV (L/min)	103	79*	79	
Volumes				
TLC (L)	5.7	8.1*	142	
RV/TLC (%)	42	42	101	
D$_{LCO}$ (mL/min/mm Hg)	27	26	96	

Comments and Questions

This 56-year-old man had a 4-year history of progressive dyspnea on exertion. He reported a productive morning cough and occasional wheezing. He had a 30 pack-year history of cigarette smoking. Coarse inspiratory and expiratory wheezes and rhonchi were heard. The chest radiograph was normal. Arterial blood gas tests at rest showed an O_2 saturation of 93%, PaO_2 of 64 mm Hg, PaCO_2 of 33 mm Hg, and pH 7.52.

1. How would you classify these data?
2. Are there any concerns you have about these data?
3. Are there other data you would like to have?

CASE 7

Answers

1. There is a mild degree of airway obstruction with a positive bronchodilator response (17%, 300 mL) to bronchodilator. The normal DLCO is not compatible with an extensive degree of emphysema. Likewise, although he has large lung volume, the normal RV/TLC ratio indicates no air trapping, also making emphysema unlikely.

2. Note that the patient was hyperventilating (low Pa_{CO_2} and increased pH) when the arterial sample was drawn.

3. To rule out emphysema, a mechanics study was done (see below). Note that despite the hyperinflation, the lung recoil is normal and the MFSR curve is to the right of the normal range, indicating that airway disease (chronic bronchitis) was the cause of the low expiratory flows. Pulmonary resistance (Rpulm) was high (5.0 cm H_2O/L/s), CL_{stat} was normal (0.250 L/cm H_2O), and CL_{dyn} was low (0.133 L/cm H_2O).

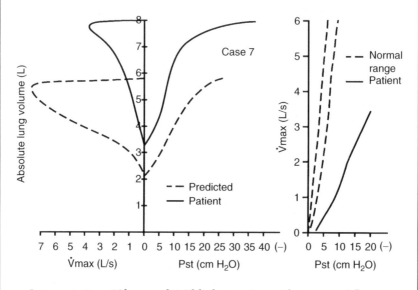

Interpretation: "Abnormal. Mild obstruction with improved flows after bronchodilator, large lung volumes but no air trapping, and normal DLCO. The MFSR curve is shifted to the right, indicating an airway predominant process."

CASE 8

36 y F Wt 211 lb (95.5 kg) Ht 63 in. (160 cm) BMI 37.3 kg/m²	Normal	Observed	% Predicted
Spirometry			
FVC (L)	3.57	1.90*	53
FEV$_1$ (L)	3.02	0.72*	24
FEV$_1$/FVC (%)	85	38*	
FEF$_{25-75}$ (L/s)	3.1	0.8*	26
MVV (L/min)	100	58*	58
Volumes			
TLC (L)	5.20	4.91	94
RV/TLC (%)	30	61*	
D$_{LCO}$ (mL/min/mm Hg)	24	11*	46

Comments and Questions

This 36-year-old woman had noted progressive shortness of breath during the past 6 years. She was a nonsmoker and had no history of asthma or a family history of lung disease. The chest radiograph revealed diffuse interstitial infiltrates. There was no response to bronchodilator.

1. What is your impression based on the above data?
2. Are there aspects of the data that are unusual?
3. Are there additional tests that might be informative?

CASE 8

Answers

1. This is a puzzling case. Obstruction is reflected in the flow–volume curve contour and the very low FEV_1, and FEV_1/FVC ratio and the increased RV/TLC. The TLC is not increased, which is unusual with this degree of obstruction. The low DLCO and the chest radiograph suggest a possible parenchymal process.

2. Lung mechanics testing was performed. Resistance was increased threefold, whereas CL_{stat} was reduced to 56% of predicted and CL_{dyn} to 30% predicted. The graphic data emphasize the lack of hyperinflation, the low maximal expiratory flows, and the relatively normal lung recoil curve. The resulting MFSR curve is consistent with extensive airway disease.

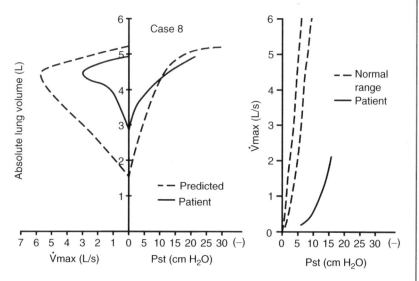

3. A lung biopsy helped with the diagnosis of lymphangioleiomyomatosis. In this case, despite the severe obstruction, there was no increase in either the TLC or CL_{stat}, a very unusual situation, which often occurs in this disease (see Case 5, page 138).

   Interpretation: "Abnormal. Very severe obstruction with air trapping and moderately reduced DLCO. The MFSR curve is shifted to the right, indicating an airway predominant process."

CASE 9

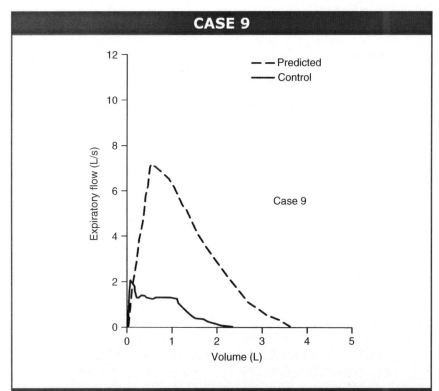

76 y   M   Wt 170 lb (77 kg)   Ht 66 in. (168 cm)   BMI 27.3 kg/m^2

Spirometry	Normal	Observed	% Predicted
FVC (L)	3.69	2.44*	66
FEV$_1$ (L)	2.83	1.33*	47
FEV$_1$/FVC (%)	77	55*	
FEF$_{25-75}$ (L/s)	2.6	0.7*	
MVV (L/min)	112	30*	27

Questions

1. What is your estimate of the degree of limitation?

2. What is causing the limitation?

3. Is there anything unusual about the test data?

4. Is there anything unusual about the flow–volume curve?

5. Is there any other test that you would order?

CASE 9

Answers

1. There is a moderately severe degree of expiratory flow limitation.

2. On the basis of the test data, the limitation is obstructive.

3. The reduced MVV at 27% predicted is lower than expected with an FEV$_1$ of 47% predicted. In our laboratory, if the MVV is less than 30× the FEV$_1$, it is interpreted as suggesting (1) muscle weakness, (2) central airway obstruction, or (3) poor patient performance. In this case, the technicians noted that the patient gave a good effort.

4. The flow–volume curve has reduced flows with a plateau in flow at about 1.3 L/s over the upper 50% of the FVC. That is typical of a central airway lesion.

5. The test that should be ordered is an inspiratory flow–volume loop. The expiratory curve and the corresponding inspiratory loop are reproduced in the figure below as the solid lines. If inspiratory flows are disproportionately reduced, usually compared at the midpoint of the vital capacity, it suggests variable extrathoracic (upper airway) obstruction. In this case, the expiratory flows are lower, suggesting that the point of flow limitation is intrathoracic.

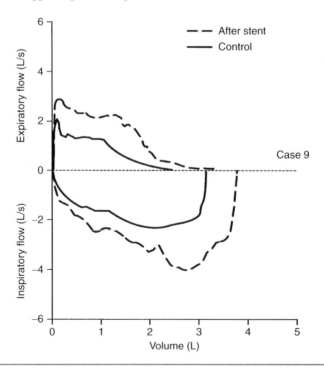

The patient was found to have granulomatosis with polyangiitis (formerly called Wegener granulomatosis). Bronchoscopy showed narrowing of both mainstem bronchi and several lobar bronchi, causing the characteristic abnormality in the flow–volume loop.

With the patient under general anesthesia, the left mainstem bronchus and bronchus intermedius were dilated, and stents were placed in both. The right mainstem bronchus was also dilated. The dashed flow–volume loop in the figure above was obtained 1 month after this procedure, and although the flows are not normal, they are much improved.

Interpretation: "Abnormal. Moderate obstruction with reduced vital capacity. A restrictive process cannot be ruled out without measurement of lung volumes. The reduced MVV raises a question of upper airway obstruction, muscle weakness, or poor performance. Inspiratory flows are relatively preserved, suggesting that the airflow limitation is predominantly intrathoracic (lower airways)."

CASE 10

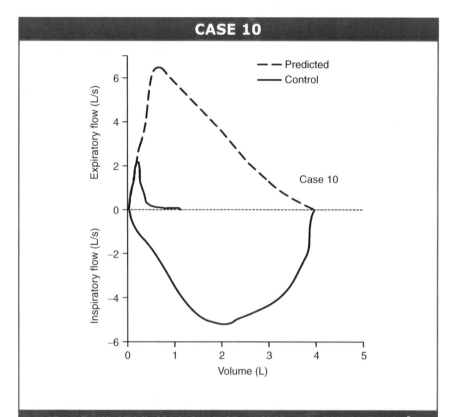

43 y   F   Wt 134 lb (61 kg)   Ht 66 in. (168 cm)   BMI 21.6 kg/m²

	Normal	Observed	% Predicted
Spirometry			
FVC (L)	3.71	1.22*	33
FEV$_1$ (L)	3.05	0.51*	17
FEV$_1$/FVC (%)	82	42*	
FEF$_{25-75}$ (L/s)	2.8	0.1*	
MVV (L/min)	111	40*	36
Volumes			
TLC (L)	5.34	6.07	114
RV/TLC (%)	31	32	103
D$_{LCO}$ (mL/min/mm Hg)	24	23	96

Comments and Questions

The inspiratory loop was obtained after a slow expiration to RV. This slow vital capacity was used to compute the RV/TLC ratio. This 43-year-old woman with a 16 pack-year smoking history had the recent onset of chest discomfort, shortness of breath, and wheezing after a viral-like illness, 3 weeks before this study.

1. What features of the control flow–volume loop are unusual?
2. Are any features of the function data unusual?
3. What might be the patient's problem?
4. Is there a procedure you might request?

CASE 10

Answers

1. The striking features of the control flow–volume loop are as follows:

a. The marked reduction in expiratory flows and volume with reasonably normal inspiratory flows and volumes—suggesting a variable intrathoracic lesion

b. The marked difference between the expiratory FVC (1.2 L) and the inspiratory vital capacity (4.0 L)

2. The spirometric values are typical of severe obstruction. An unusual finding is the normal DLco with this degree of obstruction, but that occurs in the absence of emphysema.

3. The sudden onset of this degree of obstruction and the marked difference in the inspiratory and expiratory flows and volumes suggest a major airway lesion.

4. The appropriate procedure would be chest imaging, such as standard chest radiography or CT, followed by bronchoscopy.

The patient had an abnormal chest radiograph with hilar enlargement, and bronchoscopy revealed a large squamous carcinoma nearly occluding the intrathoracic trachea (A). It was managed with laser therapy; the symptoms and the second flow–volume loop improved (B). Subsequent thoracic radiation and chemotherapy led to disappearance of the tumor, and the third spirometry was normal including inspiratory flows.

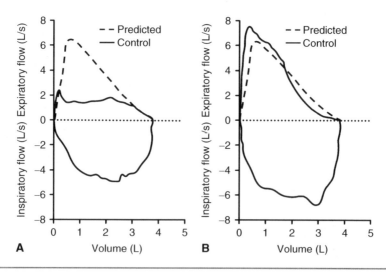

Interpretation: "Abnormal: Very severe obstruction and markedly reduced expiratory vital capacity with normal lung volumes and DLCO. The normal inspiratory flows and inspiratory vital capacity, with markedly reduced expiratory vital capacity and flows, suggest a variable intrathoracic (central airway) obstruction."

CASE 11

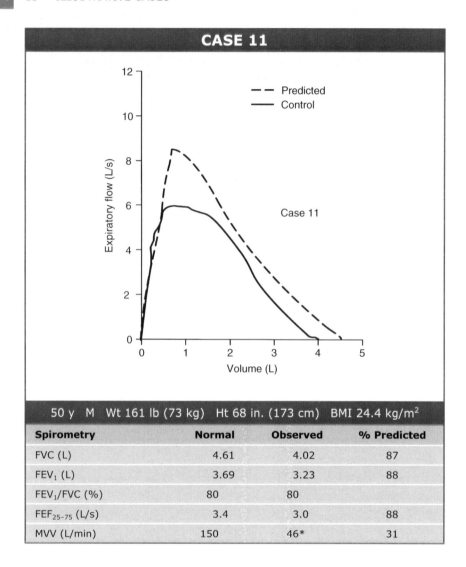

50 y M Wt 161 lb (73 kg) Ht 68 in. (173 cm) BMI 24.4 kg/m²			
Spirometry	**Normal**	**Observed**	**% Predicted**
FVC (L)	4.61	4.02	87
FEV$_1$ (L)	3.69	3.23	88
FEV$_1$/FVC (%)	80	80	
FEF$_{25-75}$ (L/s)	3.4	3.0	88
MVV (L/min)	150	46*	31

Comments and Questions

This patient complained of dyspnea on climbing stairs. He was a non-smoker. Results of cardiac examination were negative. Auscultation revealed some decrease in breath sounds. Nineteen years previously, he had had bulbar poliomyelitis, from which he recovered completely. He reported no clinical improvement after he was given a bronchodilator.

1. What is your interpretation?
2. Is there any other procedure you would order?

CASE 11

Answers

1. The flow–volume curve and spirometry results are normal. How-ever, there is a considerable reduction in the MVV. This might reflect a major airway lesion, a neuromuscular problem, or sub-maximal patient performance.

2. Because the technician thought the patient made a maximal effort on the MVV, you should order an inspiratory flow–volume curve or maximal respiratory pressures or both. This first was obtained (shown below) and indicated that the patient had severe variable extrathoracic (upper airway) obstruction with inspiratory flows less than 1 L/s. An otorhinolaryngologic examination revealed to-tal paralysis of the right vocal cord and partial paralysis of the left, resulting in an orifice-like constriction during inspiration.

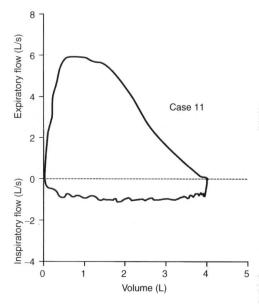

The tip-off to the diagnosis was the unexplained reduction in the MVV with what seemed to be a good effort. On the basis of the FEV_1, you would expect the MVV to be greater than 97 L/min (3.23×30). Thus, there is a striking reduction. If the inspiratory flow–volume loop were normal, you would order maximal respiratory pressures.

Interpretation: "Abnormal. MVV is severely reduced out of pro-portion to the FEV_1. Spirometry is otherwise normal. Inspiratory flows are severely reduced, consistent with variable extrathoracic (upper airway) obstruction."

CASE 12

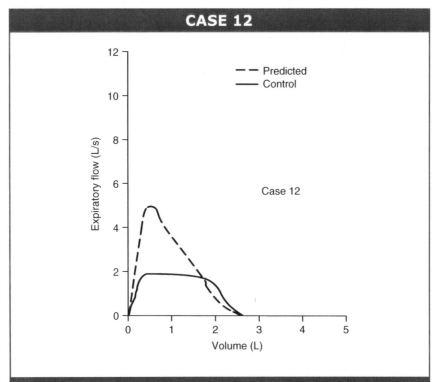

64 y F Wt 142 lb (64 kg) Ht 60 in. (152 cm) BMI 27.7 kg/m²

Spirometry	Normal	Observed	% Predicted	Postdilator
FVC (L)	2.60	2.76	106	2.70
FEV$_1$ (L)	2.13	1.84	86	1.85
FEV$_1$/FVC (%)	82	67	82	69
FEF$_{25-75}$ (L/s)	2.2	2	91	
MVV (L/min)	87	27*	31	

Comment and Question

This nonsmoker complained of the gradual onset over 5 years of dyspnea on exertion, often associated with noisy breathing.

1. What is your preliminary diagnosis, and how would you proceed?

CASE 12

Answer

1. The history, shape of the flow–volume curve, and isolated reduction in MVV suggest a "major airway lesion." A flow–volume loop (including inspiratory flows) should be obtained, which is shown in the figure below.

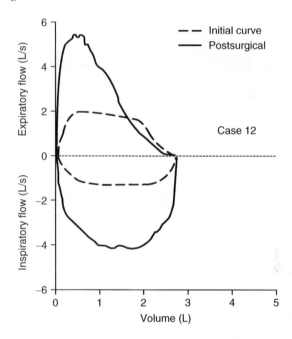

The patient had an idiopathic subglottic stenosis leading to the pattern of a fixed major airway lesion. The stricture was surgically removed, and the postoperative flow–volume loop was normal.

Interpretation: "Abnormal. MVV is markedly reduced. Although numerical results from spirometry are otherwise normal, maximal expiratory and inspiratory flows are similarly reduced in a pattern consistent with a fixed airway obstruction."

CASE 13

Comments and Questions

This patient is 62-year-old man with a body mass index (BMI) of 35 kg/m^2. He is a loud snorer with stable coronary disease.

1. How would you interpret this test?
2. Is there an unusual feature?
3. How is it relevant?

62 y Ht 188.5 cm (74 in.) Wt 124.5 kg (275 lb) BMI 35.0 kg/m^2						
	Predicted	Normal	Control	Percent Predicted	Postdilator	Percent Change
Spirometry						
FVC (L)	5.53	4.69	5.08	92	5.53	+9
FEV$_1$ (L)	4.21	3.53	4.12	98	4.11	0
FEV$_1$/FVC (%)	76.2	67.0	81.2		74.3	−9
D$_{LCO}$ (mL/min/mm Hg)	29.7	21.7	29.8	100		

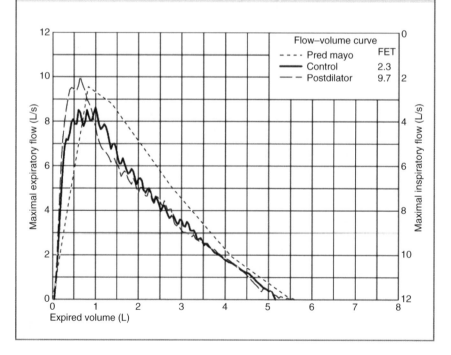

CASE 13

Answers

1. Numerical results of spirometry and D$_{LCO}$ are normal.

2. The flow–volume curve has a "sawtooth pattern."

3. This pattern, with sawtooth-shaped oscillations that have a higher frequency than occurs with coughing, is thought to be caused by oscillations of redundant tissue in the upper airways. This is seen in people who snore. Among patients with this pattern, sleep apnea is seen about twice as frequently as in those who do not demonstrate this pattern. It is worth noting as information to the clinician for possible referral for sleep consultation if clinically appropriate.

   Interpretation: "Abnormal. Numerical results of spirometry and D$_{LCO}$ are normal, and there is no response to bronchodilator. However, the sawtooth configuration of the flow–volume curve indicates redundant tissue in the upper airway. This correlates with snoring and may be predictive of obstructive sleep apnea."

CASE 14

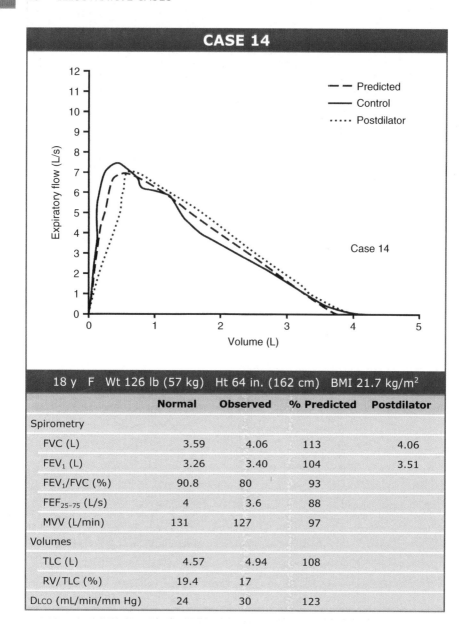

18 y F Wt 126 lb (57 kg) Ht 64 in. (162 cm) BMI 21.7 kg/m²				
	Normal	**Observed**	**% Predicted**	**Postdilator**
Spirometry				
FVC (L)	3.59	4.06	113	4.06
FEV$_1$ (L)	3.26	3.40	104	3.51
FEV$_1$/FVC (%)	90.8	80	93	
FEF$_{25-75}$ (L/s)	4	3.6	88	
MVV (L/min)	131	127	97	
Volumes				
TLC (L)	4.57	4.94	108	
RV/TLC (%)	19.4	17		
D$_{LCO}$ (mL/min/mm Hg)	24	30	123	

Questions

1. What is your interpretation?
2. The patient had a history of intermittent "chest colds" that typically last 4 to 6 weeks with some wheezing. He has responded in the past to courses of antibiotics or prednisone. Is there anything else that should be done?

CASE 14

Answers

1. The test is normal. Note the high-normal DLCO. This may be a subtle sign of underlying asthma.
2. Because of the history, you probably ordered a methacholine challenge test. The test was strongly positive after one breath of 25 mg/mL methacholine.

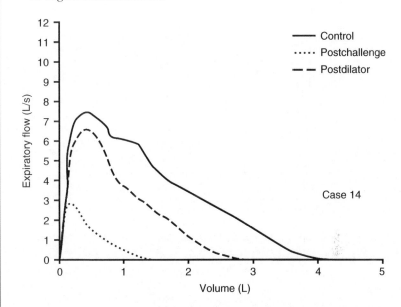

This case illustrates the importance of considering the reactivity of the airways at the time of testing. When the first test was done, the airways were fully dilated and there was no response to bronchodilator. Hence, methacholine was needed to confirm the diagnosis. In some situations, the airways may be constricted such that a bronchodilator will have a larger effect. In this case, the control FEV$_1$/FVC ratio was 80%, during the challenge, with a 67% reduction in FEV$_1$ the ratio was still 76%. This shows that the ratio does not always detect airway obstruction.

Interpretation: "Baseline spirometry, lung volumes, and DLCO are normal with no immediate response to bronchodilator. Methacholine challenge is positive after one breath of 25 mg/mL methacholine. Flows improve toward baseline after bronchodilator."

CASE 15

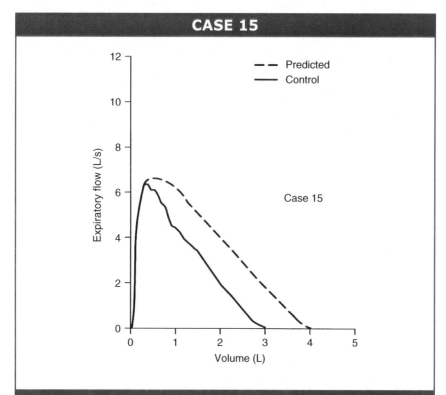

29 y F Wt 284 lb (129 kg) Ht 65 in. (165 cm) BMI 47.4 kg/m²			
	Normal	**Observed**	**% Predicted**
Spirometry			
FVC (L)	3.94	3.06*	78
FEV$_1$ (L)	3.34	2.64*	79
FEV$_1$/FVC (%)	85	86	
FEF$_{25-75}$ (L/s)	3.4	2.8	85
MVV (L/min)	120	90	75
Volumes			
TLC (L)	5.18	4.23	82
RV/TLC (%)	24	28	117
D$_{LCO}$ (mL/min/mm Hg)	25	24	96

Questions

1. Is there any ventilatory limitation?
2. On the basis of the given data, what diagnosis would you give?
3. Is there anything unusual about this patient?
4. The patient had smoked 8 cigarettes daily since age 20, 3.6 pack-years. She reported recurrent episodes of bronchitis with wheezing and breathlessness, sometimes treated with antibiotics or steroids or both. Is there any other test you would order?

CASE 15

Answers

1. The control flow–volume curve shows a small reduction in vital capacity with relatively normal flows, consistent with a mild ventilatory limitation.

2. The proportionate reductions in FVC and FEV_1, with normal TLC and FEV_1/FVC ratio, and a normal DLCO indicate a *nonspecific pattern* (see Section 3E).

3. The patient is obese with a BMI of 47.4 kg/m^2 (normal, <25).

4. On the basis of the history, a methacholine challenge test is a reasonable procedure to order because many patients with asthma are diagnosed as having bronchitis.

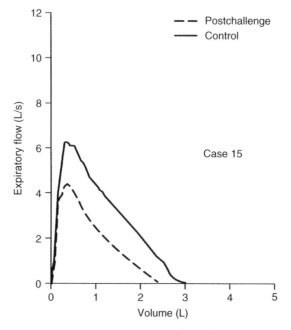

As shown in the figure, the patient has reactive airways with reduced flows after methacholine. The FEV_1 decreased by 21%.

The diagnosis now becomes "mild ventilatory limitation with reactive airways, likely due to asthma." Obesity may contribute, both by a modest effect on lung volumes and flows and perhaps by increased prevalence of airway reactivity among obese persons.

Interpretation: "Abnormal. FVC and FEV_1 are mildly reduced in a nonspecific pattern with normal TLC and FEV_1/FVC ratio. DLCO is normal. Methacholine challenge is positive."

CASE 16

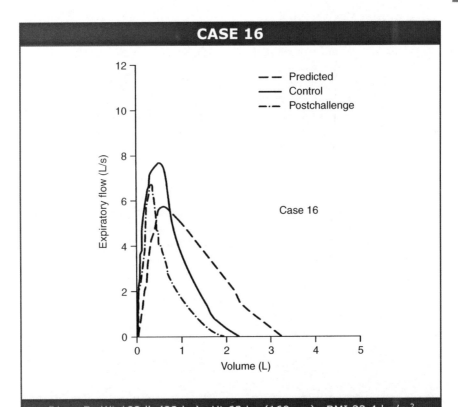

| 51 y | F | Wt 182 lb (83 kg) | Ht 63 in. (160 cm) | BMI 32.4 kg/m² |

	Normal	Observed	% Predicted	Postchallenge
Spirometry				
FVC (L)	3.24	2.38*	73	1.98 (−17%)
FEV₁ (L)	2.67	1.96*	73	1.55 (−21%)
FEV₁/FVC (%)	82	83		78
FEF₂₅₋₇₅ (L/s)	2.6	2.1	80	
MVV (L/min)	101	83	82	
Volumes				
TLC (L)	4.9	4.06	83	
RV/TLC (%)	34	33	97	
DLCO (mL/min/mm Hg)	22	21	95	

Comments

This 51-year-old woman had rheumatoid arthritis treated with low-dose prednisone. She had never smoked. Because of a history of an allergic re-action to a medication that produced mild dyspnea and cough, a metha-choline challenge was ordered.

The control study fits our definition of mild *nonspecific pattern* (see Section 3E) with mildly reduced FEV_1 and FVC and normal TLC and FEV_1/FVC ratio. The normal DLCO does not suggest a parenchymal or vascular problem, such as fibrosis, even though the flow–volume curve is rather steep. The patient is obese with a BMI of 32.4 kg/m^2, perhaps explaining the nonspecific abnormality.

Despite the normal FEV_1/FVC ratio, the patient has reactive airways with a 21% decrease in the FEV_1 after methacholine, associated with cough and some chest tightness. Thus, in this patient, the *nonspecific pattern* is associated with both obesity and asthma.

Interpretation: "Abnormal. FVC and FEV_1 are mildly reduced in a non-specific pattern with normal TLC and FEV_1/FVC ratio. DLCO is normal. Methacholine challenge is positive."

CASE 17

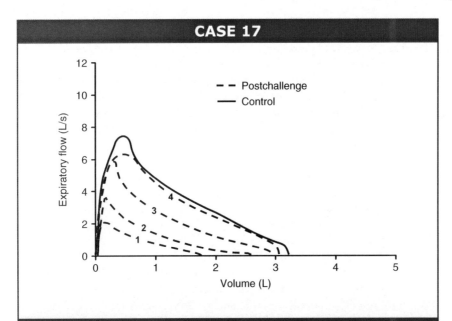

14 y   F   Wt 110 lb (50 kg)   Ht 64 in. (162 cm)   BMI 19.1 kg/m²

	Normal	Observed	% Predicted
Spirometry			
FVC (L)	3.28	3.28	100
FEV_1 (L)	2.9	2.93	101
FEV_1/FVC (%)	88	89	
FEF_{25-75} (L/s)	3.5	3.1	88
MVV (L/min)	116	117	101
Volumes			
TLC (L)	4.5	4.3	96
RV/TLC (%)	19	21	
D_{LCO} (mL/min/mm Hg)	23	23	100

Comments

This 14-year-old student is referred for evaluation of respiratory symptoms during and after soccer practice and games.

The baseline data are all normal. Because of the patient's history of intermittent wheezing and shortness of breath, a methacholine challenge was performed. The patient inhaled five breaths of the highest concentration of methacholine and her flows promptly decreased (curve 1), and the FEV_1 decreased by 62%. As repeated FVCs were obtained, the degree of bronchospasm progressively decreased, and eventually, the FEV_1 was reduced by only 14%, which is usually considered a negative test result. However, in this situation, it seems clear that the patient has hyperreactive airways. In this case, the effort of inhaling to TLC decreased the degree of bronchoconstriction, which can occur during a methacholine challenge, although this is an extreme example. The more typical behavior in a challenge is shown in Figure 5-5.

Also note the terminal portion of the control flow–volume curve. At approximately 3.2 L exhaled volume, the flow decreases precipitously to zero. As shown in Figure 2-6E, such a curve can be a normal variant, as in this case. With bronchoconstriction, this feature is lost, but it is seen again as the bronchoconstriction subsides.

Interpretation: "Indeterminate methacholine challenge. Baseline spirometry, lung volumes, and D_{LCO} are normal. After methacholine, there was an initial 62% decrease in FEV_1, which improved on subsequent efforts to the reported value. This does not meet the usual criterion for a positive challenge, but likely indicates airway hyperresponsiveness."

CASE 18

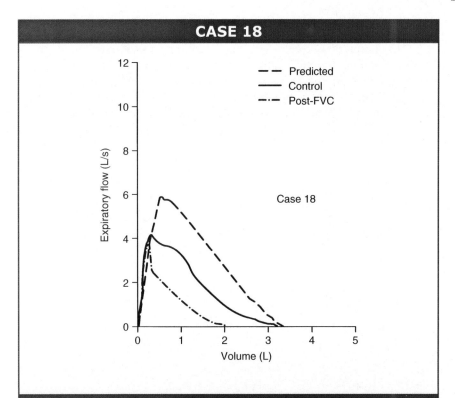

42 y F Wt 152 lb (69 kg) Ht 62 in. (157 cm) BMI 28 kg/m^2				
	Normal	**Observed**	**% Predicted**	**Post-FVC**
Spirometry				
FVC (L)	3.32	3.34	101	2.11*
FEV$_1$ (L)	2.81	2.16*	77	1.46*
FEV$_1$/FVC (%)	85	65*		
FEF$_{25-75}$ (L/s)	5.9	4.2	71	
MVV (L/min)	106	41*	39	
Volumes				
TLC (L)	4.69	4.26	91	
RV/TLC (%)	1.37	0.92	67	
D$_{LCO}$ (mL/min/mm Hg)	23	18	77	

Comments

The control flow–volume curve and data are consistent with mild airway obstruction. After the control FVC maneuver, however, audible wheezing developed and the post-FVC curve was obtained. FEV_1 was reduced by 32%. This is an example of FVC-induced bronchoconstriction, which occasionally occurs in patients with hyperreactive airways, such as in asthma. The MVV was measured after the FVC maneuver and is reduced because of the induced bronchospasm.

Interpretation: "Baseline spirometry is normal. After repeated maneuvers, the FEV_1 decreased by 32%, indicating 'FVC-induced bronchospasm' a manifestation of airways hyperresponsiveness."

CASE 19

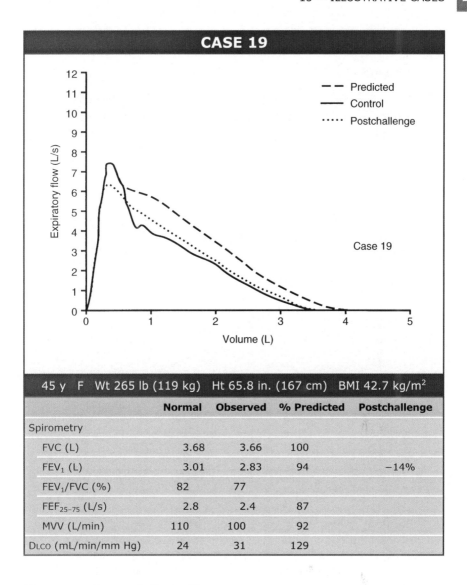

45 y F Wt 265 lb (119 kg) Ht 65.8 in. (167 cm) BMI 42.7 kg/m²				
	Normal	**Observed**	**% Predicted**	**Postchallenge**
Spirometry				
FVC (L)	3.68	3.66	100	
FEV$_1$ (L)	3.01	2.83	94	−14%
FEV$_1$/FVC (%)	82	77		
FEF$_{25-75}$ (L/s)	2.8	2.4	87	
MVV (L/min)	110	100	92	
D$_{LCO}$ (mL/min/mm Hg)	24	31	129	

Comments and Questions

This 45-year-old woman was being treated for hypertension and reported cough and wheezing with exertion. Physical examination was normal except for a blood pressure of 160/96 mm Hg. None of her medications was causing her cough. Note the negative methacholine challenge study.

1. What may be important in the data above?

2. Would you order any additional studies?

CASE 19

Answers

1. The patient is obese with a BMI of 42.7 kg/m². Obesity likely explains the increased DLCO because the challenge was negative for asthma.

2. An exercise study was ordered, and flow–volume loops were obtained. Both at rest and during exercise, as shown below, the patient breathed very near RV and on the expiratory limb of her maximal flow–volume curve.

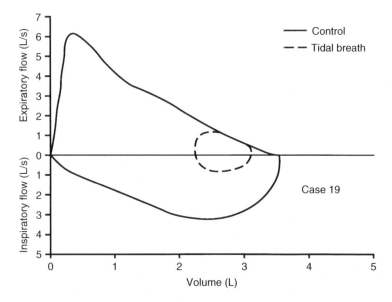

Breathing on the flow–volume curve often occurs in obese patients and produces expiratory wheezing caused by compression of the airways. Try breathing near RV and you may also wheeze. We term this *pseudoasthma*, and it is usually associated with obesity.

Interpretation: "Negative methacholine challenge. Baseline spirometry and DLCO are normal. The decrease in FEV₁ after methacholine is consistent with normal airways responsiveness. Tidal breathing during exercise shows breathing near RV and expiratory flow limitation during most of the expiratory phase."

CASE 20

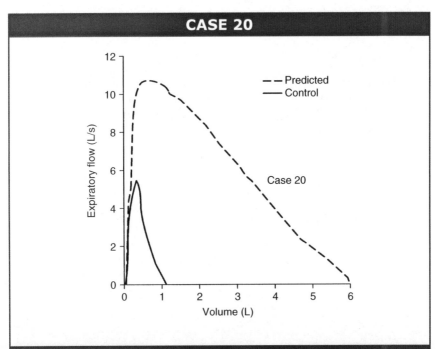

30 y   M   Wt 151 lb (68 kg)   Ht 73 in. (186 cm)   BMI 19.7 kg/m²

	Normal	Observed	% Predicted
Spirometry			
FVC (L)	6.01	1.12*	19
FEV₁ (L)	4.89	1.04*	21
FEV₁/FVC (%)	81	93	
FEF₂₅₋₇₅ (L/s)	4.6	2.2*	48
MVV (L/min)	190	81*	43
Volumes			
TLC (L)	7.45	2.09*	28
RV/TLC (%)	19	44*	232
D$_{LCO}$ (mL/min/mm Hg)	35	9*	26

Questions

1. What is your initial impression of the flow–volume curve?
2. Do the data confirm your initial impression?
3. Could obesity or a severe chest wall deformity produce these results?

CASE 20

Answers

1. The initial impression is of very severe ventilatory limitation on a restrictive basis because of the marked decreases in the TLC and FVC and the steep slope of the flow–volume curve (roughly 7L/s/L). In addition, the FEV_1/FVC ratio is high.

2. The very low TLC supports a restrictive process as the cause of the limitation. In addition, the markedly reduced D$_{LCO}$ suggests disease of the lung parenchyma. Indeed, this man had severe interstitial fibrosis of unknown cause. He also had cor pulmonale. His oxygen saturation at rest was 95%, and it decreased to 85% with mild stair climbing.

3. Although extreme obesity can reduce the TLC, it probably rarely does to this extent. In addition, a normal to increased D$_{LCO}$ might be expected in obesity. Similarly, a severe chest deformity should not be associated with this degree of reduction in the D$_{LCO}$.

   Interpretation: "Abnormal. A pulmonary parenchymal restrictive process is indicated by the very severe reductions in lung volumes and associated very severe reduction in D$_{LCO}$."

CASE 21

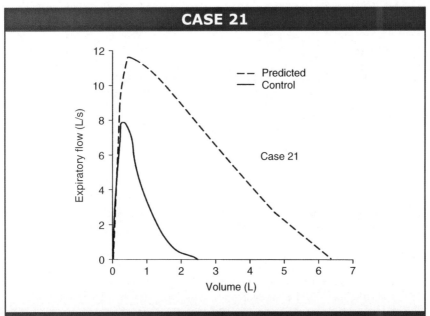

39 y M Wt 170 lb (77 kg) Arm span 79 in. (200 cm) BMI 19.3 kg/m²			
	Normal	**Observed**	**% Predicted**
Spirometry			
FVC (L)	6.32	2.37*	38
FEV$_1$ (L)	5	1.94*	39
FEV$_1$/FVC (%)	79	82	
FEF$_{25-75}$ (L/s)	4.4	2.6*	59
MVV (L/min)	186	121*	65
Volumes			
TLC (L)	7.94	3.62*	46
RV/TLC (%)	20	33	165
D$_{LCO}$ (mL/min/mm Hg)	39	19*	50

Questions

1. How do you classify the flow–volume curve?
2. What is your interpretation after reviewing the test results?
3. What is the diagnosis?

CASE 21

Answers

1. The flow–volume curve can be described as showing severe ventilatory limitation, and the slope of the curve suggests a restrictive component.

2. The severely reduced TLC confirms the presence of a restrictive defect. In addition, the moderately reduced DLCO suggests a parenchymal abnormality. Therefore, this is a severe ventilatory limitation on the basis of a restrictive process with an impaired diffusing capacity suggesting a parenchymal abnormality.

3. Note that the patient's arm span was used to predict his normal values. The patient has severe idiopathic scoliosis with areas of compressed lung. Use of the measured height would have underestimated the severity of his problem, as seen below.

The second flow–volume curve below shows the patient's curve plotted against the predicted curve for his actual height of 167.6 cm. Now the FVC is 54% of predicted versus 38%, and the FEV$_1$ shows a similar difference. The point is that the technicians should measure the arm span and use it to predict the normal values for patients with spinal deformities. The arm span should also be used on patients who cannot stand up straight or who are in a wheelchair.

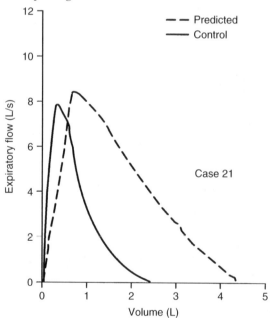

Interpretation: "Severe restriction with moderately reduced DLCO, consistent with a pulmonary parenchymal process (arm span used for calculating reference values)."

CASE 22

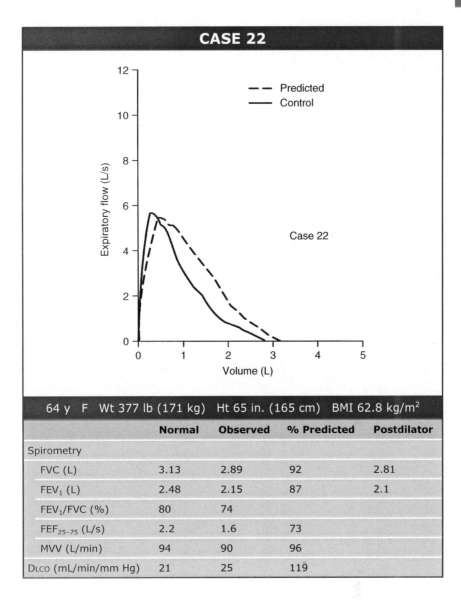

64 y F Wt 377 lb (171 kg) Ht 65 in. (165 cm) BMI 62.8 kg/m²				
	Normal	**Observed**	**% Predicted**	**Postdilator**
Spirometry				
FVC (L)	3.13	2.89	92	2.81
FEV$_1$ (L)	2.48	2.15	87	2.1
FEV$_1$/FVC (%)	80	74		
FEF$_{25-75}$ (L/s)	2.2	1.6	73	
MVV (L/min)	94	90	96	
D$_{LCO}$ (mL/min/mm Hg)	21	25	119	

Question

1. How would you interpret this test?

CASE 22

Answer

1. The contour of the flow–volume curve may suggest borderline airway obstruction but is actually normal at this age, as is the FEV_1/FVC ratio. The normal FVC makes restriction very unlikely. The patient's high BMI might lead you to expect an abnormality of spirometry, but that is not invariably the case. Note the mild elevation in the D_{LCO}.

   This case illustrates that even in older patients, morbid obesity (the BMI is 62.8 kg/m^2) does not necessarily have an adverse effect on lung function.

   Interpretation: "Normal spirometry and D_{LCO} with no immediate response to bronchodilator."

CASE 23

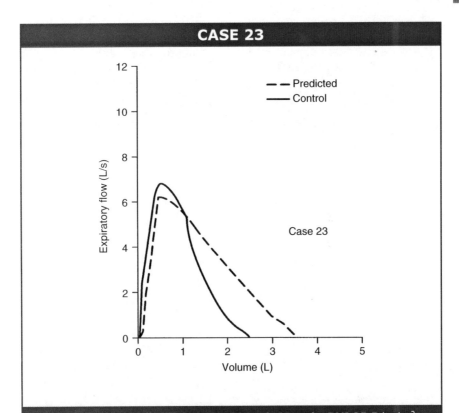

49 y   F   Wt 158 lb (72 kg)   Ht 66 in. (168 cm)   BMI 25.5 kg/m^2

	Normal	Observed	% Predicted
Spirometry			
FVC (L)	3.55	2.43	68
FEV$_1$ (L)	2.89	2.20	76
FEV$_1$/FVC (%)	81	91	
FEF$_{25-75}$ (L/s)	2.7	3.3	123
MVV (L/min)	106	92	87
Volumes			
TLC (L)	5.31	4.39	83
RV/TLC (%)	33	36	109
D$_{LCO}$ (mL/min/mm Hg)	23	14*	61

Comments and Questions

The patient complained of dyspnea climbing one flight of stairs. She had never smoked. She had some skin thickening and joint stiffness and pain.

1. What does the flow–volume curve suggest?
2. Considering the test results, what is your final interpretation? (Note that during the past 3 years, the TLC, FVC, and D_{LCO} have gradually declined.)

CASE 23

Answers

1. The lost area under the normal curve suggests mild ventilatory limitation. The rather steep slope of the flow–volume curve suggests either a restrictive process or a nonspecific process, depending on the TLC.

2. The low-normal TLC does not quite qualify as a restrictive pattern, but it may raise your suspicion. The best interpretation is that of a mild nonspecific ventilatory limitation associated with a reduced diffusing capacity.

   The patient has scleroderma with minimal interstitial fibrosis shown by radiography, which explains the reduced D_{LCO} and probably the steep slope of the flow–volume curve. The fibrosis and the chest skin changes of scleroderma can reduce the TLC, though not significantly in this case.

   Interpretation: "Abnormal. D_{LCO} is mildly to moderately reduced, consistent with the pulmonary parenchymal or vascular process. The low-normal lung volumes raise a question of a restrictive process."

CASE 24

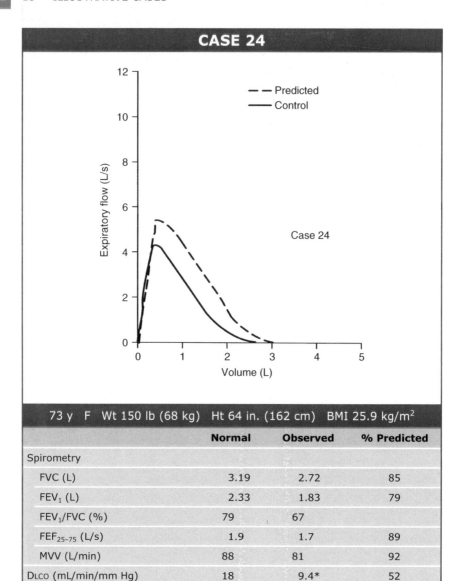

73 y   F   Wt 150 lb (68 kg)   Ht 64 in. (162 cm)   BMI 25.9 kg/m²

	Normal	Observed	% Predicted
Spirometry			
FVC (L)	3.19	2.72	85
FEV$_1$ (L)	2.33	1.83	79
FEV$_1$/FVC (%)	79	67	
FEF$_{25-75}$ (L/s)	1.9	1.7	89
MVV (L/min)	88	81	92
D$_{LCO}$ (mL/min/mm Hg)	18	9.4*	52

Comments and Questions

This 73-year-old woman complained of cough for 2 months. The cough had begun after a flu-like illness. She was a nonsmoker. She denied wheezing and dyspnea. On examination, her lungs were clear. She had a grade 4/6 harsh precordial holosystolic murmur.

1. How would you interpret this test? (She did not show any response to inhaled bronchodilator.)
2. What might be the cause of her problem?

CASE 24

Answers

1. On the basis of the area comparison, there is suggestion of a mild ventilatory limitation of a nonspecific nature, the FEV$_1$/FVC ratio being in the normal range. The moderately reduced diffusing capacity is consistent with a restrictive process caused by a lung parenchymal abnormality, but because there is not a measure of TLC, this cannot be confirmed.

2. The loud murmur was the important clue. Her chest radiograph showed an interstitial pattern (easily confused with fibrosis), small bilateral pleural effusions, and an enlarged heart. An echocardiogram showed a reduced left ventricular ejection fraction and severe mitral regurgitation. With therapy for the congestive heart failure, her cough disappeared, and she lost 12 lb. The flow–volume curve below was then obtained. It was totally normal, and the diffusing capacity also normalized.

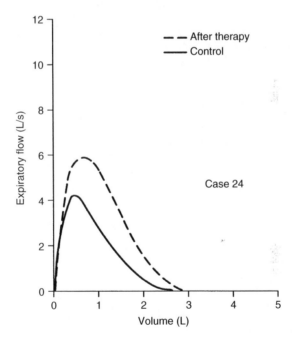

Congestive heart failure can present with cough or dyspnea as isolated complaints. The pulmonary function test can mimic a restrictive process caused by congested lymphatics and perivascular and peribronchial edema. In other cases, the spirometry and flow–volume curve may suggest obstruction. This can be quite marked and present as "cardiac asthma."

Interpretation: "Abnormal. D$_{LCO}$ is moderately reduced, consistent with a pulmonary vascular or parenchymal process. Spirometry results are in the low-normal range. Subsequent spirometry and D$_{LCO}$ are normal."

CASE 25

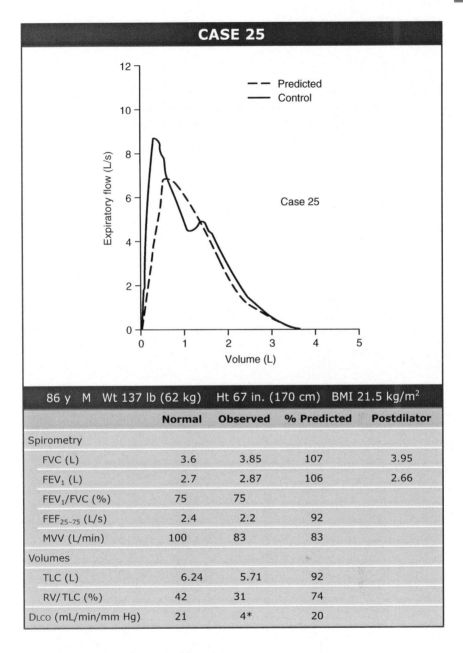

86 y M Wt 137 lb (62 kg) Ht 67 in. (170 cm) BMI 21.5 kg/m²				
	Normal	**Observed**	**% Predicted**	**Postdilator**
Spirometry				
FVC (L)	3.6	3.85	107	3.95
FEV₁ (L)	2.7	2.87	106	2.66
FEV₁/FVC (%)	75	75		
FEF₂₅₋₇₅ (L/s)	2.4	2.2	92	
MVV (L/min)	100	83	83	
Volumes				
TLC (L)	6.24	5.71	92	
RV/TLC (%)	42	31	74	
DLCO (mL/min/mm Hg)	21	4*	20	

Comment and Questions

This is a case of an isolated reduction in the DLCO.

1. What might be the cause of this finding?
2. Is there any significance to the contour of the flow–volume curve?

CASE 25

Answers

1. A poor effort or equipment problems could cause this low DLCO value. However, the test was repeated on a different unit and was not changed. The patient was not anemic, but severe anemia could contribute to a reduced DLCO. The tests showed no evidence of emphysema. The chest radiograph did show an extensive fine interstitial infiltrate thought to represent metastatic cancer. The mildly reduced RV/TLC ratio might reflect an early restrictive process, but essentially the volumes and spirometry results are normal.

2. The notch in the flow–volume curve was not seen on other efforts and is of no significance.

Interpretation: "Abnormal. DLCO is very severely reduced, consistent with a pulmonary vascular or parenchymal disorder. Spirometry and lung volumes are normal."

CASE 26

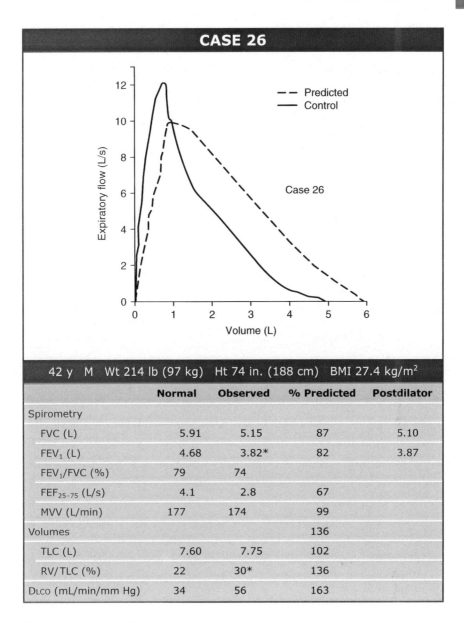

42 y M Wt 214 lb (97 kg) Ht 74 in. (188 cm) BMI 27.4 kg/m²				
	Normal	**Observed**	**% Predicted**	**Postdilator**
Spirometry				
FVC (L)	5.91	5.15	87	5.10
FEV$_1$ (L)	4.68	3.82*	82	3.87
FEV$_1$/FVC (%)	79	74		
FEF$_{25-75}$ (L/s)	4.1	2.8	67	
MVV (L/min)	177	174	99	
Volumes			136	
TLC (L)	7.60	7.75	102	
RV/TLC (%)	22	30*	136	
D$_{LCO}$ (mL/min/mm Hg)	34	56	163	

Comment and Questions

The patient is a smoker.

1. How would you interpret this study?
2. What is particularly unusual, and what might be the cause?

CASE 26

Answers

1. The flow–volume curve suggests mild airway obstruction. The reduced FEV_1 is consistent with this impression, even with the normal FEV_1/FVC ratio.

2. The unusual feature is the remarkable increase in the D_{LCO}. Such an increase can occur in asthma, obesity, non–resting state, pulmonary hemorrhage, and polycythemia. The patient had an atrial septal defect with a significant left-to-right shunt. This produced an increased pulmonary capillary blood volume and, hence, the high D_{LCO}.

   Interpretation: "Abnormal. D_{LCO} is markedly increased. In the absence of asthma, obesity, or non–resting state, this may be due to polycythemia, left-to-right shunt, or pulmonary hemorrhage. Spirometry shows a mild nonspecific reduction in FEV_1 with normal FEV_1/FVC ratio and TLC. There is no immediate response to bronchodilator."

CASE 27

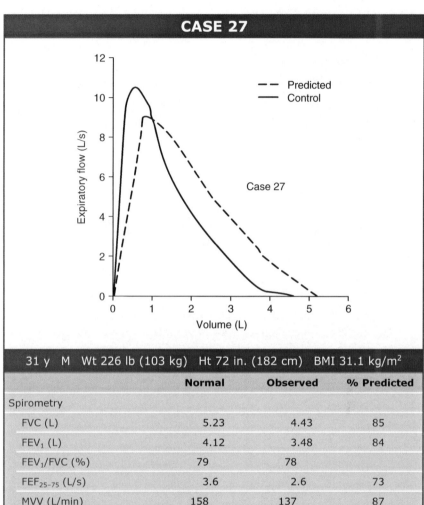

31 y M Wt 226 lb (103 kg) Ht 72 in. (182 cm) BMI 31.1 kg/m²			
	Normal	**Observed**	**% Predicted**
Spirometry			
FVC (L)	5.23	4.43	85
FEV$_1$ (L)	4.12	3.48	84
FEV$_1$/FVC (%)	79	78	
FEF$_{25-75}$ (L/s)	3.6	2.6	73
MVV (L/min)	158	137	87
Volumes			
TLC (L)	7.11	7.38	104
RV/TLC (%)	27	36*	
D$_{LCO}$ (mL/min/mm Hg)	33	26	79
O$_2$ saturation (%)			
Rest	96	90*	
Exercise	96	85*	

Questions

1. Is there anything in the data to explain the patient's desaturation?
2. Can you rule out some possible causes?

CASE 27

Answers

1. Nothing in the data indicates the cause of the patient's desaturation. The mild increase in the RV/TLC ratio is not helpful.

2. The flow–volume curve shows borderline ventilatory limitation, but nothing indicates the cause of the problem. The TLC and D_{LCO} effectively rule out lung parenchymal disease. The patient is mildly obese (BMI is 31.1 kg/m^2), but the weight is not severe enough to cause this problem.

The patient had advanced liver disease with small intrathoracic right-to-left shunts, causing the desaturation. The patient exhibited orthodeoxia, namely, the saturation decreased when he went from the recumbent to the standing position. He underwent liver transplantation, which was successful, and the desaturation was abolished.

Impression: "Abnormal. Oxygen saturation is reduced at rest and falls further during exercise. Spirometry, lung volumes, and D_{LCO} are normal, other than a slightly increased RV that may result from very mild obstruction or chest wall limitation."

CASE 28

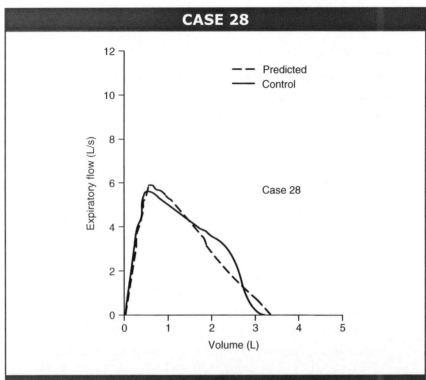

45 y F Wt 131 lb (60 kg) Ht 62 in. (157 cm) BMI 24.3 kg/m²				
Spirometry	**Normal**	**Observed**	**% Predicted**	**Postdilator**
FVC (L)	3.44	3.96	115	4.0
FEV$_1$ (L)	2.84	2.98	105	
FEV$_1$/FVC (%)	82	75		
FEF$_{25-75}$ (L/s)	2.7	3.51	130	
MVV (L/min)	106	122	115	

Comments and Questions

A 45-year-old woman had noted dyspnea when hurrying on the level or when climbing stairs for the past 1 to 2 years. She also had slight weakness of both the upper extremities.

1. What is your interpretation of this test?
2. Is there any other test you would order?

CASE 28

Answers

1. The spirometry is normal, including MVV and the flow–volume curve.

2. Did you order maximal respiratory pressure measurements? Unexplained dyspnea and slight muscle weakness should alert you to the possibility of a neuromuscular disorder.

	Normal	Observed	Percent of Normal
PImax (cm H_2O)	−70	−26*	37
PEmax (cm H_2O)	135	90*	67

The maximal respiratory pressures are both reduced, with inspiratory more than expiratory. Neurologic examination and electromyography confirmed a diagnosis of amyotrophic lateral sclerosis. This is an example of dyspnea caused by muscle weakness appearing at a time when spirometry results, including the MVV, were still normal.

Interpretation: "Abnormal. Maximal respiratory pressures are reduced, consistent with neuromuscular weakness (particularly, inspiratory pressure). Spirometry is otherwise normal, including MVV."

CASE 29

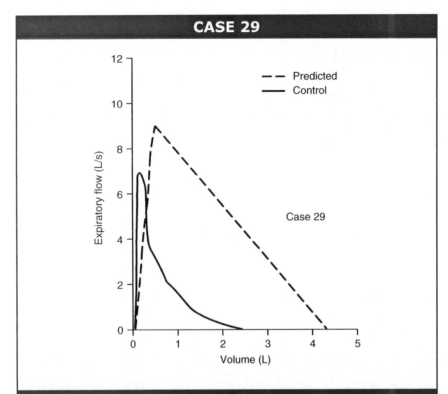

68 y M Wt 224 lb (102 kg) Ht 74 in. (188 cm) BMI 28.9 kg/m²			
	Normal	**Observed**	**% Predicted**
Spirometry			
FVC (L)	4.36	2.43*	56
FEV_1 (L)	3.05	1.59*	52
FEV_1/FVC (%)	70	66	
FEF_{25-75} (L/s)	2.7	0.7*	26
MVV (L/min)	117	87*	75
Volumes			
TLC (L)	7.84	4.95*	63
RV/TLC (%)	44	51	116
D_{LCO} (mL/min/mm Hg)	36	28	78

Comments and Questions

1. This 68-year-old man had recently noted becoming short of breath when lying down. He slept best in a recliner. He denied dyspnea while walking or climbing stairs. He had been a heavy smoker but quit 15 years ago.
2. What is your initial impression of the flow–volume curve?
3. Do the test results agree with your initial assessment?
4. Are there any other tests you might order?

CASE 29

Answers

1. The flow–volume curve suggests moderate ventilatory limitation that, on the basis of the reduced TLC and FVC, appears to be restrictive in nature. Shape of the flow–volume curve and the low-normal FEV$_1$/FVC ratio raises the question of an obstructive component as well.

2. The test results do not provide a diagnosis. The patient's BMI of 28.9 kg/m^2 is not sufficient to explain the restrictive component as being due to obesity. The relatively normal DLCO argues against interstitial lung disease.

3. The patient's intolerance for lying flat suggested diaphragmatic paralysis. The physician ordered diaphragmatic ultrasound, which confirmed that impression. The physician also ordered a supine flow–volume curve. Note the marked reduction of volumes and flows obtained in the supine posture.

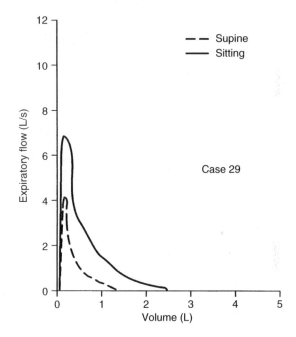

The physician also ordered maximal respiratory pressure measurements:

PEmax was 215 cm H$_2$O (normal, 200)

PImax was −36 cm H$_2$O (normal, −103)

These data are consistent with paralysis of the diaphragm. In summary, this patient's symptoms were attributable to restriction without evidence of interstitial disease. Further evaluation pointed to a form of weakness, which was eventually identified as diaphragmatic paralysis.

Interpretation: "Abnormal. A restrictive process is indicated by the mild-to-moderate reductions in TLC and FVC. There is no definite evidence of obstruction. D_{LCO} is in the low-normal range, suggesting an extraparenchymal cause of restriction. The decrease in vital capacity in the supine position and low maximal inspiratory pressure suggests inspiratory muscle (e.g., diaphragm) weakness. Maximal expiratory pressure is normal."

CASE 30

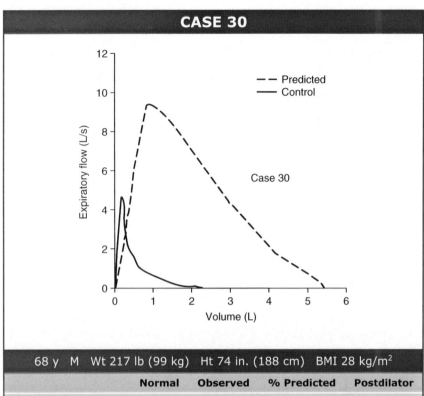

68 y M Wt 217 lb (99 kg) Ht 74 in. (188 cm) BMI 28 kg/m²				
	Normal	**Observed**	**% Predicted**	**Postdilator**
Spirometry				
FVC (L)	5.46	2.33*	43	2.2
FEV$_1$ (L)	4.10	1.17*	28	1.19
FEV$_1$/FVC (%)	75	50*		
FEF$_{25-75}$ (L/s)	3.3	0.4*	12	0.4
MVV (L/min)	145	50*	34	
Volumes				
TLC (L)	7.69	4.74*	62	
RV/TLC (%)	29	46*	159	
D$_{LCO}$ (mL/min/mm Hg)	28	17*	60	

Question

1. How would you interpret the results?

CASE 30

Answer

1. There is very severe ventilatory limitation on a mixed obstructive and restrictive basis. The restriction is reflected in the mild-to-moderate reduction in TLC. The obstruction is reflected in the very severely reduced FEV_1. The degree of obstruction is moderate (see Chapter 3, Section 3F). There is a mild-to-moderate reduction of the diffusing capacity.

The patient had obstructive lung disease and had undergone a left pneumonectomy 10 years previously for squamous cell lung cancer, causing the restrictive component. Considering this, the DLCO is relatively well preserved.

Interpretation: "Abnormal. Very severe mixed obstructive/restrictive process. Mild-to-moderate restriction is indicated by the reduction in TLC. The disproportionate reduction in FEV_1 with reduced FEV_1/FVC ratio indicates superimposed moderate obstruction. There is no immediate response to bronchodilator. DLCO is mildly to moderately reduced, consistent with a pulmonary vascular or parenchymal process or anemia."

CASE 31

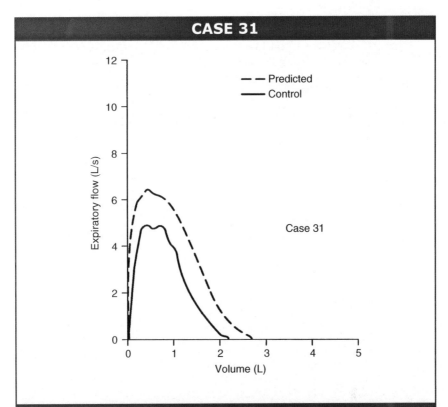

40 y   F   Wt 213 lb (97 kg)   Ht 62 in. (157 cm)   BMI 39.4 kg/m^2

	Normal	Observed	% Predicted
Spirometry			
FVC (L)	3.32	2.14*	64
FEV$_1$ (L)	2.59	1.94*	75
FEV$_1$/FVC (%)	77	90	
FEF$_{25-75}$ (L/s)	3.07	2.72	89
MVV (L/min)	107	79	74
Volumes			
TLC (L)	4.65	4.02	86
RV/TLC (%)	32	35	109

Comments and Questions

The patient gave a 4-year history of episodes of shortness of breath. Typically, she had nocturnal nonproductive coughing and awoke with dyspnea but no wheezing. Attacks would subside in 1 to 2 days, and she knew of nothing that precipitated them. She was a nonsmoker. Results of physical examination were unremarkable: Her lungs were clear, and her heart was normal.

1. What is your interpretation of this test?
2. What do you think the problem is?
3. Are there any other procedures you would order?

CASE 31

Answers

1. The proportionate reduction in the FVC and FEV_1 with a normal FEV_1/FVC ratio suggests a restrictive process. However, the normal TLC rules out restriction. Thus, she has a *nonspecific pattern*.

2. As shown previously, a normal FEV_1/FVC ratio does not rule out obstruction. Because of the nocturnal nature of the patient's symptoms, you may have suspected asthma or reflux and aspiration.

3. If you ordered a bronchodilator, you were correct. As can be seen from the flow–volume curves below, the postdilator curve is normal. The FEV_1 increased by 25%.

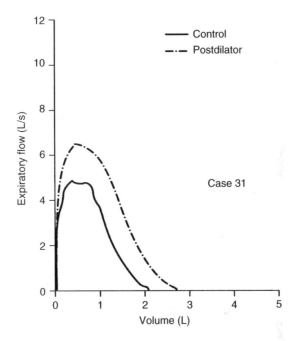

This case reinforces several points:

Not all asthmatics wheeze.

Asthma is often a nocturnal disorder.

The patient's excess weight (BMI is 39.4 kg/m²) may have contributed to the nonspecific pattern.

This is another example of the FEV_1/FVC ratio not being an infallible indicator of obstruction.

The two flow–volume curves really show a parallel shift, as is often seen in mild asthma. In these instances, the FEV_1/FVC ratio does not decrease until more severe obstruction develops.

Interpretation: "Abnormal. FVC and FEV_1 are mildly reduced in nonspecific pattern with normal TLC and FEV_1/FVC ratio. Both normalize after bronchodilator, indicating a reversible obstructive disorder."

CASE 32

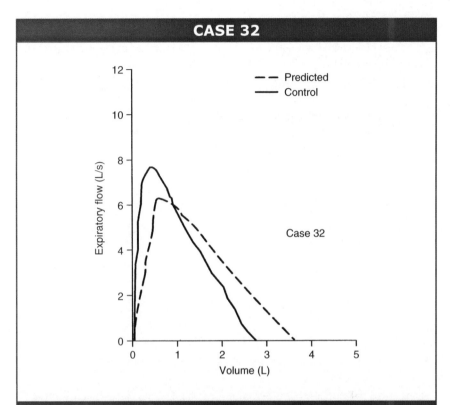

22 y F Wt 117 lb (53 kg) Ht 60 in. (152 cm) BMI 22.9 kg/m²				
	Normal	**Observed**	**% Predicted**	**Postdilator**
Spirometry				
FVC (L)	3.63	2.83*	78	2.65
FEV₁ (L)	3.21	2.58*	81	2.49
FEV₁/FVC (%)	88	92		
FEF₂₅₋₇₅ (L/s)	3.7	3.8	103	
MVV (L/min)	118	88	75	
Volumes				
TLC (L)	4.45	3.6	81	
RV/TLC (%)	18	22	122	
DLCO (mL/min/mm Hg)	24	23	93	

Comments and Questions

This 22-year-old woman was seen for a lump in her throat that interfered with swallowing and for anxiety. She noted in passing that sometimes she became short of breath, but she denied wheezing. Results of physical examination were negative.

1. How would you interpret the flow–volume curve and test data?
2. Is there any other procedure you would order?

CASE 32

Answers

1. The mildly reduced FVC and FEV_1 with normal TLC and FEV_1/ FVC ratio indicate a nonspecific pattern. There is no bronchodilator response and a normal DLCO. Airway resistance was measured and was normal.

2. Because the results of cardiac examination were normal and the cause of her dyspnea was unknown, a methacholine challenge test was ordered. The curve after five breaths of 25 mg/mL methacholine is shown below. There was a 55% decrease in FEV_1 associated with chest tightness and mild dyspnea similar to what the patient had been experiencing.

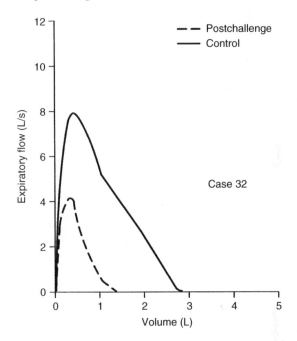

An interesting feature is the parallel shift in the postmethacholine curve, resulting in an FEV_1/FVC ratio that was 90% despite the severe bronchoconstriction. In addition, the measurement of airway resistance during the initial part of the study failed to detect any abnormality. The slightly increased slope of the control curve and the low-normal TLC might raise the question of mild pulmonary fibrosis, but of course, the normal DLCO argues against this. In fact, this is an example of occult asthma characterized mainly by a decrease in the FEV_1 and FVC and some increase in the slope of the flow–volume curve, that is, a *nonspecific pattern*. It underscores the fallacy of using FEV_1/FVC ratio as the sole criterion for obstructive disorders.

Interpretation: "Baseline pulmonary function shows mild nonspecific reductions in FVC and FEV_1 with normal TLC and FEV_1/FVC ratio. D_{LCO} is normal. There was no immediate response to bronchodilator. Subsequent methacholine challenge was positive."

CASE 33

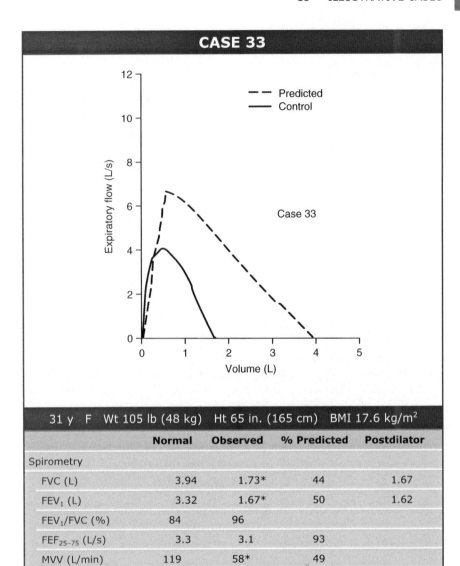

31 y F Wt 105 lb (48 kg) Ht 65 in. (165 cm) BMI 17.6 kg/m²				
	Normal	**Observed**	**% Predicted**	**Postdilator**
Spirometry				
FVC (L)	3.94	1.73*	44	1.67
FEV$_1$ (L)	3.32	1.67*	50	1.62
FEV$_1$/FVC (%)	84	96		
FEF$_{25-75}$ (L/s)	3.3	3.1	93	
MVV (L/min)	119	58*	49	
Volumes				
TLC (L)	5.26	5.43	103	
RV/TLC (%)	25	68*		
D$_{LCO}$ (mL/min/mm Hg)	25	29	114	

Questions

1. How would you interpret this test?

2. Do the flow–volume curve and test data suggest the need for other tests?

CASE 33

Answers

1. There is significant ventilatory limitation (i.e., loss of area under the flow–volume curve). The curve is steep, but the normal TLC and diffusing capacity rule out a pulmonary parenchymal restrictive process. At this point, this case can be classified as a *nonspecific pattern*.

2. There are no findings to suggest a major airway lesion. However, another possible cause of such a pattern is a neuromuscular problem. Maximal respiratory pressures should be determined to assess respiratory muscle strength.

The values follow:

	Normal	Patient	Percent of Normal
PImax (cm H_2O)	−88	−26	30
PEmax (cm H_2O)	154	35	23

The patient has severe amyotrophic lateral sclerosis. The muscle weakness led to the decreased FVC, FEV_1, and MVV and the increased RV/TLC ratio. Surprisingly, a normal TLC was maintained. Compare this case with Case 28, a less severe case of muscle weakness.

Interpretation: "Abnormal. FVC and FEV_1 are moderately to severely reduced in a nonspecific pattern with normal TLC and FEV_1/FVC ratio. The low maximal respiratory pressures indicate muscle weakness or poor performance."

CASE 34

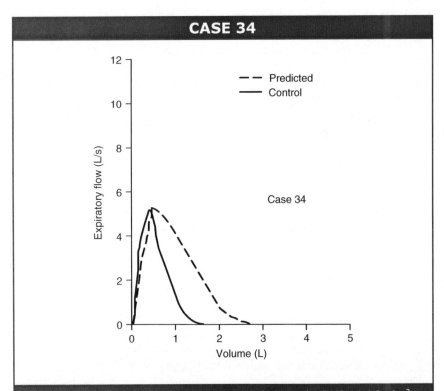

72 y F Wt 249 lb (113 kg) Ht 63 in. (160 cm) BMI 44.1 kg/m²			
	Normal	**Observed**	**% Predicted**
Spirometry			
FVC (L)	2.75	1.56*	57
FEV$_1$ (L)	2.18	1.34*	62
FEV$_1$/FVC (%)	79	86	
FEF$_{25-75}$ (L/s)	2	1.7	
MVV (L/min)	86	53*	62
Volumes			
TLC (L)	4.88	3.77*	77
RV/TLC (%)	44	51	116
D$_{LCO}$ (mL/min/mm Hg)	20	16	79

Question

1. What is your interpretation of the results in this 72-year-old nonsmoking woman?

CASE 34

Answer

1. This is a restrictive process based on the mild reduction in TLC. The disproportionate moderate reduction in FVC indicates a complex restrictive process. The normal DLCO argues against a severe parenchymal process causing the restriction. Thus, the restriction is extrapulmonary and most likely due to obesity (BMI is 44.1 kg/m^2). This case contrasts with Case 22 (page 177), in which even greater obesity caused no reduction in the FVC and presumably no change in the TLC. On average, obesity causes a reduction of 5% in FVC for each 5 unit increase in BMI, but the effect is highly variable. It may be marked, as in this case, or negligible, as in Case 22.

Interpretation: "Abnormal. Complex restrictive process. A restrictive process is indicated by the mild reduction in TLC. The disproportionate reduction in FVC relative to TLC suggests an additional process, which may include chest wall limitation (possibly related to obesity), muscle weakness, poor performance, or occult obstruction. DLCO is in the low-normal range, arguing against a significant parenchymal restrictive process."

CASE 35

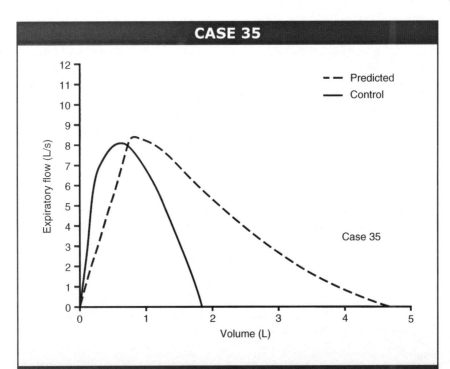

77 y M Wt 150 lb (68 kg) Ht 72 in. (182 cm) BMI 20.5 kg/m²			
	Normal	**Observed**	**% Predicted**
Spirometry			
FVC (L)	4.72	1.83*	39
FEV$_1$ (L)	3.53	1.83*	52
FEV$_1$/FVC (%)	75	99.7	
FEF$_{25-75}$ (L/s)	2.8	6.1	216
MVV (L/min)	126	93*	74
Volumes			
TLC (L)	7.16	4.75*	66
RV/TLC (%)	34	61*	179
D$_{LCO}$ (mL/min/mm Hg)	25	15*	60

Comments

FVC is severely reduced but TLC is only mildly reduced, a complex restrictive pattern. There is no evidence of obstruction and no response to bronchodilator. Oxygen saturation is normal at rest and during exercise. The shape of the flow–volume curve, reduced TLC and DLCO, and high FEV$_1$/FVC ratio are all consistent with a parenchymal restrictive process, such as fibrosis. However, the disproportionate reduction in FVC and the normal oximetry are atypical. The patient had congestive heart failure with bilateral pleural effusions. Congestive heart failure can mimic pulmonary fibrosis. Contrast this case with Case 24, page 182. Congestive heart failure may present with a variety of pulmonary function patterns including either restriction or obstruction or both. Restrictive cases may be simple or complex. To review the causes of restriction, see Chapter 12.

Interpretation: "Abnormal. Complex restrictive process. A pulmonary parenchymal restrictive process is indicated by the mild reduction in TLC and associated mild-to-moderate reduction in DLCO. The disproportionate reduction FVC, a relative to TLC, suggests an additional process which may include chest wall limitation, neuromuscular weakness, poor performance, or occult obstruction."

CASE 36

Comments and Questions

This patient is a 91-year-old man with a BMI of 31 kg/m². He is a former 35 pack-year smoker with severe dyspnea.

1. Does the patient have ventilatory limitation? Is the flow–volume curve normal?
2. Does that mean his lungs are undamaged by smoking? Is there any other abnormality?
3. How should you interpret this?

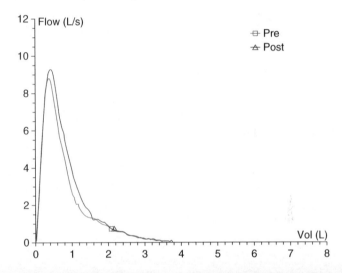

91 y Ht 170.6 cm (67 in.) Wt 90.7 kg (200 lb) BMI 31 kg/m²

	Predicted	Normal	Control	Percent Predicted	Postdilator	Percent Change
Spirometry						
FVC (L)	3.21	2.24	3.44	107	3.74	+9
FEV₁ (L)	2.34	1.55	2.05	88	2.15	+5
FEV₁/FVC (%)	73.9	57.5	59.6		57.5*	−3
Volumes						
TLC (L)	6.55	5.40	6.55	100		
RV/TLC (%)	49	58	48	97		
D$_{LCO}$ (mL/ min/mm Hg)	20.1	12.1	4.9*	24		
O₂ saturation at rest			85			

CASE 36

Answers

1. There is no definite ventilatory limitation. The FEV₁/FVC ratio is slightly abnormal after bronchodilator only. Note that the lower limit for FEV₁/FVC ratio is quite low at this age, a reflection of normal aging on lung mechanics. The flow–volume curve shows quite a bit of curvature or "scooping," but at age 91, that is not abnormal.

2. Although spirometry and lung volumes are normal, gas exchange is markedly impaired.

3. Chest radiography suggested, and CT scan confirmed, that this patient has both severe emphysema and pulmonary fibrosis. Thus, his is a case of combined pulmonary fibrosis and emphysema (CPFE). This is primarily a pulmonary parenchymal disorder, as opposed to a pulmonary vascular disorder. Loss of elastic recoil, caused by emphysema, is counterbalanced by increased elastic recoil from pulmonary fibrosis, balancing the lung mechanics to yield normal spirometry with a severe gas exchange abnormality.

Interpretation: "Abnormal. There is an isolated severe reduction in DLCO, consistent with a pulmonary vascular or parenchymal process. Spirometry and lung volumes are normal with no immediate response to bronchodilator."

CASE 37

Comment and Questions

This is a 73-year-old man with dyspnea after a lengthy hospitalization for infectious endocarditis.

1. What is the primary abnormality? How would you interpret this test?
2. Would you grade the abnormality as mild, moderate, or severe?
3. The initial interpretation was, "Mild restrictive physiology without significant bronchodilator response. Diffusing capacity, adjusted for hemoglobin, is reduced." Do you agree?

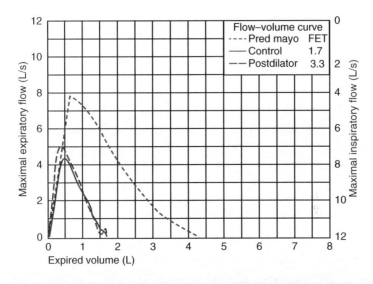

73 y   Ht 174.9 cm (69 in.)   Wt 64.4 kg (142 lb)   BMI 21 kg/m²

	Predicted	Normal	Control	Percent Predicted	Postdilator	Percent Change
Spirometry						
FVC (L)	4.24	3.40	1.63*	38	1.62*	−1
FEV₁ (L)	3.24	2.56	1.54*	48	1.47*	−5
FEV₁/FVC (%)	76.4	67.2	94.7		90.9	
Volumes						
TLC (L)	6.60	5.23	4.38*	66		
RV/TLC (%)	35.8	46.9	63*	176		
DLCO (mL/ min/mm Hg)	25.0	17.0	5.4*	22		

CASE 37

Answers

1. The patient had previous infectious endocarditis and valve replacement complicated by biventricular heart failure, pulmonary hypertension, chronic pleural thickening, residual critical illness myopathy, and suspicion of aspiration. He has a restrictive process. He fits what we have described as the "complex restrictive" pattern (see Chapter 3, Section 3H, and Chapter 14), in which TLC is reduced with a normal FEV_1/FVC ratio, but FVC is reduced further, by at least 10% predicted. In patients with this pattern, there is usually "something else" in place of, or in addition to, a typical restrictive process.

2. TLC is only mildly or moderately reduced (depending on which grading algorithm you use). In contrast, FVC is severely reduced, and DLCO is very severely reduced. This illustrates the dilemma of this pattern and the rationale for calling it "complex."

3. Calling this "mild" ignores the severe reduction in ventilatory capacity indicated by the low FVC and the very severe gas exchange abnormality indicated by the DLCO. The interpretation fails to recognize the severity of the abnormality. The patient died less than a year after the test. The interpretation also fails to grade the severity of the gas exchange abnormality. There has never been a controversy over the cut points for grading severity of abnormality of DLCO. Failing to name the severity of an abnormality of DLCO is a disservice to the ordering physician as well as the patient.

Interpretation: "Abnormal, complex restrictive disorder. A pulmonary parenchymal restrictive process is indicated by the mild reduction in TLC and associated very severe reduction in DLCO. The disproportionate severe reductions in vital capacity and FEV_1, relative to TLC, suggest an additional process, which might include chest wall limitation, muscle weakness, poor performance, or occult obstruction. There is no acute response to bronchodilator. The patient is unable to exhale for 6 seconds or more, which may contribute to the reduction in FVC."

CASE 38

Questions

1. Does this 20-year-old woman have ventilatory limitation?
2. Do the test values support your impression?
3. Is the configuration of the flow–volume curve normal?

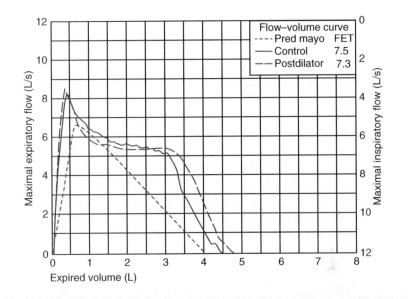

20 y Ht 170.6 cm (67 in.) Wt 90.7 kg (200 lb) BMI 31 kg/m²						
	Predicted	**Normal**	**Control**	**Percent Predicted**	**Postdilator**	**Percent Change**
Spirometry						
FVC (L)	3.99	3.25	4.47	112	4.71	+5
FEV₁ (L)	3.47	2.92	4.07	112	4.29	+5
FEV₁/FVC (%)	87.0	75.9	91.1		91.1	
DLCO (mL/ min/mm Hg)	25.0	17.0	25.4	99		
VA (mL)	4.80	3.83	4.99	104		

CASE 38

Answers

1. There is no ventilatory limitation.

2. The test values are all normal.

3. Over most of the vital capacity, flow decreases in a relatively grad-ual, steady manner. However, at 3 L of expired volume, there is a "knee" in the curve after which flow decreases more rapidly. This contour is not caused by a major airway lesion but is a normal variant that occurs mostly in young nonsmokers, espe-cially women. This patient had never smoked. This shape is due caused by the transition of the point of flow limitation moving peripherally as lung volumes decrease. The "knee" represents the lung volume at which the point of flow limitation moves to the mainstem bronchi, then moves further toward the periphery as lung volume decreases. This is called a *tracheal plateau*. It can be considered a sign of healthy peripheral airways (see Fig. 2-6H). Interestingly, this patient has cystic fibrosis with normal lung function at the time of this test. She has had some episodes of "mucous plugging" but, with aggressive care in a Cystic Fibrosis Care Center, has maintained stable function over 6 years since this test (FVC is unchanged as well).

This case also illustrates a testing rule we use in our lab. If the pa-tient is ordered to have a "full pulmonary function testing (PFT)" and has a normal spirometry and normal alveolar volume (VA), as this patient does, measurements of lung volumes are cancelled unless the provider orders a "mandatory TLC," thus saving the patient the cost of an unnecessary test. Note that VA is a measure-ment of TLC. As a single breath gas dilution test, it may underesti-mate, but rarely overestimates, TLC.

Interpretation: "Normal spirometry and D$_{LCO}$ with no immediate response to bronchodilator. The shape of the flow–volume curve is a normal variant."

CASE 39

Questions

1. What type of ventilatory limitation does this woman have? Obstruction? Restriction? Something else? How would you describe this pattern?

2. What are likely causes of this pattern?

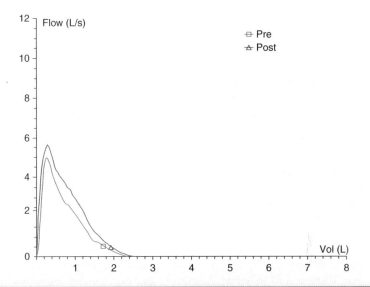

53 y Ht 164.0 cm (65 in.) Wt 144.4 kg (319 lb) BMI 54 kg/m²

	Predicted	Normal	Control	Percent Predicted	Postdilator	Percent Change
Spirometry						
FVC (L)	3.43	2.11	2.37*	69	2.51*	+6
FEV₁ (L)	2.73	2.11	1.72*	63	1.91*	+5
FEV₁/FVC (%)	80.0	68.7	72.6		76.3	
MVV (L/min)	102	69	72	71		
Volumes						
TLC (L)	5.03	4.05	4.40	87		
RV/TLC (%)	37	47	41	111		
DLCO (mL/min/mm Hg)	22.6	16.1	16.2	72		
O₂ saturation at rest			95			

CASE 39

Answers

1. She has mild reductions in both FEV_1 and FVC with a normal FEV_1/FVC ratio. This does not indicate obstruction. This fits the pattern described as PRISm (Preserved Ratio Impaired Spirometry) by the COPDGene investigators. Half of patients with this pattern have restriction, but half have a normal TLC as does this patient. So this is also concordant with the "nonspecific pattern" described in Chapter 3, Section G.

2. The majority of patients with this pattern are obese, as is this patient. Most have evidence of obstructive airway disease, such as chronic obstructive pulmonary disease (COPD) or asthma, despite the normal FEV_1/FVC ratio. Chest wall abnormalities and neuromuscular weakness are common contributing factors as well.

This 53-year-old woman has ANCA-associated vasculitis treated with steroids and immunosuppressive medications. She has cough and dyspnea and a focal right lower lobe ground-glass infiltrate. Bronchoscopy with bronchoalveolar lavage showed no evidence of opportunistic infection and no endobronchial abnormality or central airway obstruction. She is obese (with a BMI of 54 kg/m^2) and has obstructive sleep apnea. Her mild nonspecific pattern is likely related to her obesity. The ground-glass opacity may contribute to the reduction in FVC and FEV_1, but not enough to cause significant reduction in either TLC or DLCO. The normal bronchoscopy revealed no evidence of airway collapse or stricture, and although the normal MVV is encouraging, it would be worthwhile to obtain inspiratory flows at some point.

Interpretation: "Nonspecific abnormality. FVC and FEV_1 are mildly reduced in nonspecific pattern with a normal TLC and FEV_1/FVC ratio. There is no immediate response to bronchodilator. DLCO and resting oximetry are normal. The patient was unable to exercise. Obesity may contribute to the nonspecific abnormality."

CASE 40

Annual monitoring of change in lung function can identify persons with accelerated decline due to smoking, occupational exposures, or other causes. This person has normal lung function, which is stable over 9 years of employment. The estimated rate of decline in FEV$_1$ is −17 mL/y, which is normal.

Case 40

Age: 41 y	Date	FVC	FEV$_1$	FEF max	QC flow	QC volume
	06/04/1991	4.50	3.70	12.3	A	A
	06/26/1991	4.42	3.63	11.7	B	A
	03/26/1992	4.26	3.51	10.7	B	A
	10/28/1992	4.22	3.48	11.8	A	A
	09/02/1993	4.42	3.47	12.4	A	A
	04/12/1994	4.64	3.66	10.9	A	A
	03/14/1995	4.44	3.43	11.1	A	A
	03/13/1996	4.52	3.51	12.3	C	A
	02/19/1997	4.71	3.57	12.6	A	A
	03/10/1998	4.76	3.70	15.8	A	A
	03/24/1999	4.39	3.37	11.2	B	A
	02/29/2000	4.40	3.38	10.9	C	A

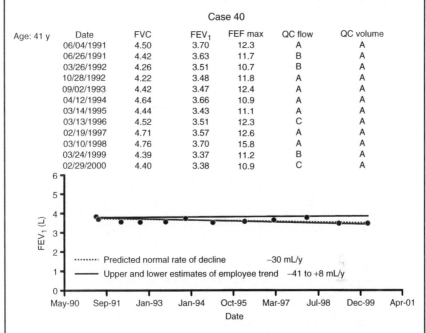

Predicted normal rate of decline   −30 mL/y

Upper and lower estimates of employee trend   −41 to +8 mL/y

(This is an actual trend report with data from individual tests. QC flow and QC volume are grades for maneuver quality.)

CASE 41

This person, a 44-year old smoker at the time of his most recent test, is in a respiratory protection program. He has had a rapid decline in lung function over 8 years. His estimated rate of decline in FEV$_1$ is -138 mL/y. Mild obstruction has developed already. He is very likely to be disabled before retirement, unless appropriate preventive measures are taken.

Case 41

Age: 44 y	Date	FVC	FEV$_1$	FEF max	QC flow	QC volume
	12/16/1991	3.54	3.07	13.3	A	A
	11/19/1992	3.62	3.16	13.0	A	A
	04/14/1994	3.42	2.86	12.4	C	B
	07/22/1996	3.35	2.81	13.7	C	C
	08/22/1997	2.50	2.26	10.9	A	A
	09/14/1998	2.59	2.39	13.6	B	B
	02/29/2000	2.10	1.95	11.4	C	C

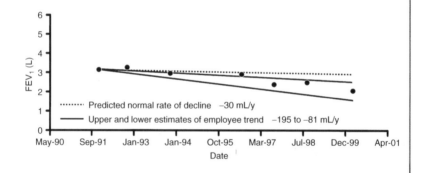

Predicted normal rate of decline -30 mL/y

Upper and lower estimates of employee trend -195 to -81 mL/y

CASE 42

More frequent monitoring may be needed for persons with labile lung function, such as those with asthma, and for persons with lung injury or lung transplantation. This trend shows gradual improvement in lung function of an employee of a chemical plant who was heavily exposed to chlorine in an industrial accident. Lung function improved rapidly during the first month after his injury, then slowly during the following 5 years.

Case 42

	Date	FVC	FEV$_1$	FEV$_1$/FVC (%)	FEF 25–75	PEF	QC flow	QC volume
Age: 41 y	04/07/98	3.78	2.94	78	2.44	13.1	A	A
Ht: 172.7 cm	02/19/97	3.51	2.73	78	2.24	12.0	A	A
Wt: 119 kg	05/07/96	3.56	2.65	74	1.93	11.9	A	A
	10/04/95	3.47	2.56	74	1.80	12.2	A	A
	02/23/95	3.47	2.62	76	2.08	10.8	B	A
	11/30/94	3.44	2.61	76	2.07	9.9	A	A
	09/01/94	3.30	2.60	79	2.25	11.4	A	A
	07/14/94	3.27	2.53	77	2.13	10.2	A	A
	06/23/94	3.32	2.58	76	2.16	11.1	A	A
	05/26/94	2.96	2.29	77	1.93	9.9	A	A
	05/12/94	2.94	2.27	77	1.84	10.7	A	A
	04/28/94	2.72	2.06	76	1.63	8.7	C	C
	04/07/94	1.67	1.27	76	0.97	5.9	B	B
	03/31/94	1.87	1.48	79	1.34	6.7	A	A
	01/26/94	3.66	2.89	79	2.61	9.9	B	A
	11/15/93	3.78	3.02	80	2.84	10.5	C	C
	12/21/92	3.90	3.09	79	2.79	10.5	A	A

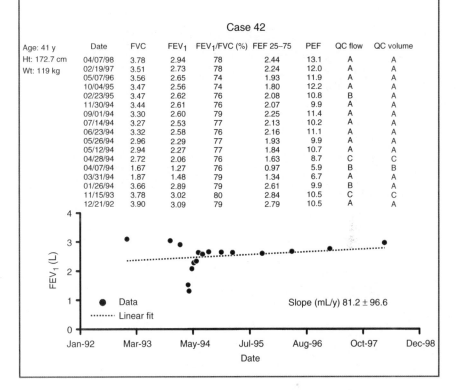

CASE 43

This trend from a patient who had lung transplantation shows gradual improvement over 2 months, then an episode of rejection, which was treated successfully 7 months after transplantation. Values indicated by an "X" were deleted from analysis because they were outliers caused by a wet flow element (see Case 45).

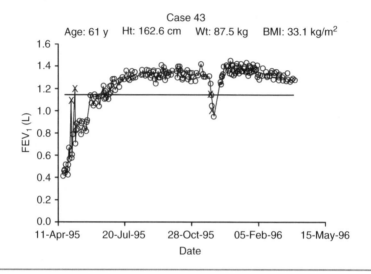

Case 43
Age: 61 y   Ht: 162.6 cm   Wt: 87.5 kg   BMI: 33.1 kg/m^2

CASE 44

This trend shows the progressive decline in function of a patient with obliterative bronchiolitis after lung transplantation.

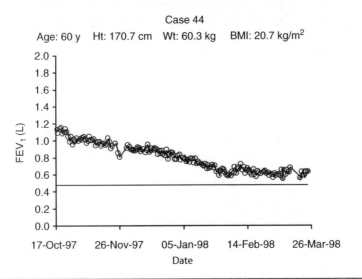

Case 44

Age: 60 y   Ht: 170.7 cm   Wt: 60.3 kg   BMI: 20.7 kg/m^2

CASE 45

This trend is highly variable with frequent "spikes" showing artifactual increases in FEV_1. These were due to the patient's use of a wet spirometer flow sensor. The moisture increases the flow resistance of the element, giving an increase in driving pressure and causing an overestimate of his FEV_1. Values indicated by an "X" were deleted from analysis because they were outliers caused by a wet flow element. After the patient was reinstructed in proper care of the spirometer, the artifact was eliminated.

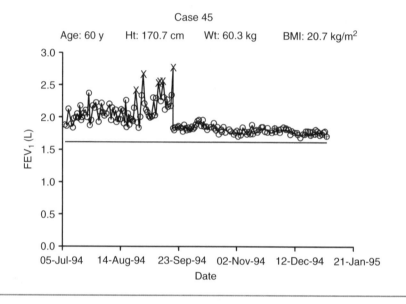

Case 45

Age: 60 y   Ht: 170.7 cm   Wt: 60.3 kg   BMI: 20.7 kg/m^2

Types of Cases

Pulmonary Function Interpretation Template

XXXX CITY

(Test performed at Mxxx Clinic Health System in XXXX City, interpreted at Mxxx Clinic Rxxxx.)

AMENDED

(Amended report) 00/00/2019.

PERFORM UNABLE

The patient was unable to perform acceptable and repeatable maneuvers, so results may underestimate true lung function.

PERFORM DIFFICULTY

The patient had difficulty performing maneuvers, so results may underestimate true lung function.

PERFORM COUGH

The patient had difficulty performing maneuvers because of coughing. This may result in underestimation of FEV_1.

NL SPIRO

Normal spirometry.

NL SPIRO and BDN

Spirometry is normal with no immediate response to bronchodilator.

NL SPIRO and DLCO

Normal spirometry and D_{LCO}.

NL SPIR and VOL and DL

Normal spirometry, lung volumes, and D_{LCO}.

TRACHEAL PLATEAU

The prominent "tracheal plateau" on the flow–volume curve is likely a normal variant.

FVC QUIT

FVC is underestimated because of premature termination of expiratory effort.

PERFORM MVV

The low MVV may be result from muscle weakness or upper airways obstruction, but more likely poor performance.

SPIRO NON

Abnormal. FVC and FEV_1 are mildly reduced in a nonspecific pattern.

BOO

Borderline obstruction.

MIO

Abnormal. Mild obstruction.

MOO

Abnormal. Moderate obstruction.

SEO

Abnormal. Severe obstruction.

VSO

Abnormal. Very severe obstruction.

SPIRO MIX

Abnormal. Mild/moderate/severe obstruction with reduced vital capacity. The low vital capacity may be caused by air trapping, but a superimposed restrictive process cannot be ruled out without measurement of lung volumes.

SPIRO AIR TRAP

Abnormal. Mild/moderate/severe obstruction with reduced vital capacity (the latter has previously been shown to be caused by air trapping, not superimposed restriction).

WEAK

MVV and maximal respiratory/inspiratory/expiratory pressure/pressures is/are reduced, consistent with muscle weakness or poor performance.
However, MVV/maximal respiratory/inspiratory/expiratory pressure/pressures is/are normal.

VETO

Inspiratory flows are reduced relative to expiratory flows, and MVV is also reduced out of proportion to FEV_1, indicating variable extrathoracic (upper airway) obstruction, muscle weakness, or poor performance.

INSP FLOW NL

Inspiratory flows are relatively preserved.

VITO

Expiratory flows are reduced relative to inspiratory flows, and the shape of the expiratory flow–volume curve suggests a central airway obstructive process.

FIXED

Inspiratory and expiratory flows are reduced, and the shape of the flow–volume curves indicates a fixed central airway obstructive process.

SAWTOOTH

The sawtooth configuration of the flow–volume curve indicates redundant tissue in the upper airway. This correlates with snoring and may be predictive of obstructive sleep apnea.

VOLS NL

with normal lung volumes.

AIR TRAP

with air trapping.

HYPER

with hyperinflation.

BDY

Flows improve after bronchodilator.

BDY COMMENT

Flows improve after bronchodilator, suggesting an element of reversible obstruction.

BD FVC

The improvement in vital capacity after bronchodilator indicates reduced air trapping.

BDY NL SPIRO

Although there is no clear evidence of obstruction, the improved flows after bronchodilator suggests a reversible obstructive process.

BD LG

There is a large improvement in flows after bronchodilator.

BDN

There is no immediate response to bronchodilator.

BDM

There is minimal improvement in flows after bronchodilator.

PERFORM BD

The apparent response to bronchodilator may indicate an element of reversible obstruction, but more likely represents improved performance.

POS MECH

Positive methacholine challenge. Baseline pulmonary function shows_____ Flows improve toward baseline after bronchodilator.

NEG MECH

Negative methacholine challenge. Baseline pulmonary function shows_____ The decrease in FEV_1 after methacholine is consistent with normal airways responsiveness.

BOR MECH

Borderline methacholine challenge. Baseline pulmonary function shows_____ The decrease in FEV_1 after methacholine does not meet the criteria for a positive challenge, but may indicate mild airway hyperresponsiveness.

POS EXERCISE

Positive exercise challenge. Baseline pulmonary function shows_____ Flows improve toward baseline after bronchodilator.

NEG EXERCISE

Negative exercise challenge. Baseline spirometry shows_____

NON SPIRO

Abnormal. FVC and FEV_1 are mildly reduced in a nonspecific pattern. The possibility of a restrictive process could be further evaluated with measurement of lung volumes, if clinically indicated.

NON

Abnormal. FVC and FEV_1 are mildly/moderately/severely reduced in a nonspecific pattern with a normal TLC, FEV_1/FVC ratio, and airways resistance.

NON OBSTRUCT

The increased airway resistance, shape of the flow–volume curve, and response to bronchodilator suggest a partly reversible obstructive process.

RESTRICT

Abnormal. A pulmonary parenchymal restrictive process is indicated by the mild/moderate/severe reductions in lung volumes and associated mild/moderate/severe reduction in DLCO (after adjustment for low hemoglobin).

COMPLEX

Complex restriction. A restrictive process is indicated by the mild/moderate/severe reduction in TLC. The disproportionate mild/moderate/severe reduction in vital capacity and FEV_1, relative to TLC, suggests an additional process, which might include chest wall limitation, muscle weakness, poor performance, or occult obstruction.

MIX

Mild/moderate/severe mixed abnormality. A restrictive process is indicated by the mild/moderate/severe reduction in TLC. The disproportionate reduction in FEV_1 and the reduced FEV_1/FVC ratio indicate superimposed mild/moderate/severe obstruction. DLCO is normal.

DLCO LOW

DLCO is mildly/moderately/severely reduced, consistent with emphysema or other pulmonary vascular or parenchymal process.

DLCO ADJ LOW

DLCO (adjusted/unadjusted for hemoglobin) is mildly/moderately/severely reduced, consistent with a pulmonary parenchymal or vascular process or anemia.

DL5

Although technically acceptable, the validity of the very low D_{LCO} is uncertain.

DL3

D_{LCO} is not reportable because of technically uncertain results.

DLCO AND OXY NL

D_{LCO} (adjusted/unadjusted for hemoglobin) and oximetry are normal.

DLCO AND OXY NLLO

D_{LCO} (adjusted/unadjusted for hemoglobin) and resting oximetry are normal. Saturation decreases during exercise.

OXY NL

Oxygen saturation is normal at rest and during exercise.

OXY NL REST

Oxygen saturation is normal at rest. The patient was unable to exercise.

OXY NLLO

Oxygen saturation is normal at rest but decreases during exercise.

OXY LOLO

Oxygen saturation is reduced at rest and decreases further during exercise.

OXY VLO

Oxygen saturation is markedly reduced at rest. Exercise was not attempted.

TACHY

Note that the patient was tachycardic at rest.

OTHER NL

Lung volumes, spirometry, inspiratory flows, maximal inspiratory/expiratory/respiratory pressure/pressures, D_{LCO}, resting oximetry, resting, and exercise oximetry are normal.

COMPARE NC

Compared with 00/00/20XX, there has been no change.

COMPARE

Compared with 00/00/20XX,
TLC, spirometry, FVC, FEV_1, pre-bronchodilator FVC and FEV_1, postbronchodilator FVC and FEV_1, inspiratory flows, maximal inspiratory/expiratory/respiratory pressure/pressures, D_{LCO}, resting oximetry, resting, and exercise oximetry
are/is
increased/unchanged/decreased.
has/have
improved/not changed/declined.
But/however/and
TLC, spirometry, FVC, FEV_1, pre-bronchodilator FVC and FEV_1, postbronchodilator FVC and FEV_1, inspiratory flows, maximal inspiratory/expiratory/respiratory pressure/pressures, D_{LCO}, resting oximetry, resting, and exercise oximetry
are/is
increased/unchanged/decreased.
has/have
improved/not changed/declined.
The increase/decrease in
TLC, spirometry, FVC, FEV_1, prebronchodilator FVC and FEV_1, postbronchodilator FVC and FEV_1, inspiratory flows, maximal inspiratory/expiratory/respiratory pressure/pressures, D_{LCO}, resting oximetry, resting, and exercise oximetry is/are within the variability of the measurement.

HE VERSUS PLETH

The apparent increase/reduction in TLC is likely due to differences in technique (helium dilution vs. plethysmography).

Index

Note: Page numbers followed by *f* indicate a figure; *t* following a page number indicates tabular material.